LLEWELLYN'S

COMPLETE BOOK OF
ESSENTIAL OILS

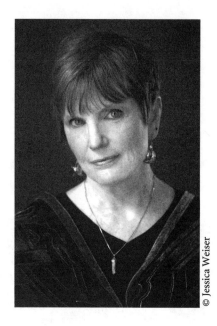

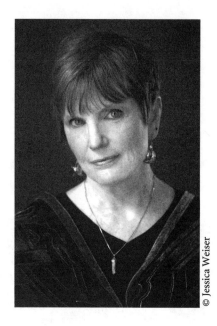© Jessica Weiser

About the Author

Sandra Kynes is a Reiki practitioner and a member of the Bards, Ovates & Druids. She likes to develop creative ways to explore the world and integrate them into her spiritual path, which serves as the basis for her books. Sandra has lived in New York City, Europe, England, and now coastal New England. She loves connecting with nature through gardening, hiking, bird watching, and ocean kayaking. Visit her website at www.kynes.net.

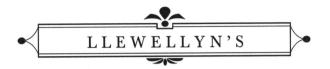

LLEWELLYN'S

COMPLETE BOOK OF

ESSENTIAL OILS

How to Blend, Diffuse, Create Remedies,
and Use in Everyday Life

SANDRA KYNES

LLEWELLYN PUBLICATIONS
Woodbury, Minnesota

FIRST EDITION
First Printing, 2019

Cover design by Shannon McKuhen
Interior art by the Llewellyn Art Department

Llewellyn Publishing is a registered trademark of Llewellyn Worldwide Ltd.

Library of Congress Cataloging-in-Publication Data

Names: Kynes, Sandra, author.
Title: Llewellyn's complete book of essential oils : how to blend, diffuse,
   create remedies, and use in everyday life / by Sandra Kynes.
Other titles: Complete book of essential oils
Description: First edition. | Woodbury, MN : Llewellyn Publications, a
   division of Llewellyn Worldwide Ltd., 2019. | Series: Llewellyn's complete
   book series ; 13 | Includes bibliographical references and index.
Identifiers: LCCN 2019015997 (print) | LCCN 2019016656 (ebook) | ISBN
   9780738757100 (ebook) | ISBN 9780738756875 (alk. paper)
Subjects: LCSH: Essences and essential oils. | Formulas, recipes, etc. |
   Deodorization. | Self-care, Health.
Classification: LCC TP958 (ebook) | LCC TP958 .K96 2019 (print) | DDC
   661/.806—dc23
LC record available at https://lccn.loc.gov/2019015997

Llewellyn Worldwide Ltd. does not participate in, endorse, or have any authority or responsibility concerning private business transactions between our authors and the public.

All mail addressed to the author is forwarded but the publisher cannot, unless specifically instructed by the author, give out an address or phone number.

Any internet references contained in this work are current at publication time, but the publisher cannot guarantee that a specific location will continue to be maintained. Please refer to the publisher's website for links to authors' websites and other sources.

Llewellyn Publications
A Division of Llewellyn Worldwide Ltd.
2143 Wooddale Drive
Woodbury, MN 55125-2989
www.llewellyn.com
Printed in the United States of America

Also by Sandra Kynes

365 Days of Crystal Magic (2018)

Crystal Magic (2017)

Plant Magic (2017)

Bird Magic (2016)

The Herb Gardener's Essential Guide (2016)

Star Magic (2015)

Llewellyn's Complete Book of Correspondences (2013)

Mixing Essential Oils for Magic (2013)

Change at Hand (2009)

Sea Magic (2008)

Your Altar (2007)

Whispers from the Woods (2006)

A Year of Ritual (2004)

Gemstone Feng Shui (2002)

Forthcoming Books

Magical Symbols & Alphabets (2020)

Herbal Remedies for Beginners

Tree Magic

Contents

Contents

• • • • • • • •

• • • • • • • •

Contents

· · · · · · · ·

PART SEVEN: CARRIER OILS AND OTHER INGREDIENTS   243

• • • • • • •

Contents

Figures

Tables

· · · · · · ·

Disclaimer

The information in this book is not intended to replace medical advice. Essential oils should not be taken internally without the supervision of a physician or trained healthcare provider. Do not use essential oils for conditions that are already being treated without the advice of your doctor. When using remedies to treat minor problems, contact your doctor if a problem becomes prolonged or escalates.

INTRODUCTION

Scents stimulate, inspire, and enchant us. Because our sense of smell is so closely linked with memory and emotion, scent and the power of place are deeply intertwined. Some of my most vivid childhood memories are linked with my grandmother's house, which was full of plants and big old furniture. Most of all, I remember the smells. With her potpourris, gardens, and big kitchen, her house was a wonderland of fragrance.

Like many people, I became interested in essential oils because of their enticing scents. The fact that I could mix them myself to make my own perfume was an exciting prospect. I am a perpetual student. I love learning and studying, which I do mostly on my own, supplemented with the occasional class or workshop. As I experimented with essential oils, I found that combining some of them did not work as well as I had hoped, so I went in search of information.

I found plenty of recipes, which were fun for a while, but I wanted to know more and understand what I was doing. This coincided with my interest in making potpourri, which often involves the use of essential oils. I jumped at the chance to take a Saturday afternoon workshop where I hoped to learn more about mixing essential oils. Although it was a good class, it didn't fulfill all my expectations, and making headway with essential oils was slow.

I wanted to understand why certain oils work well together and others do not. I wanted to know how to go about making intelligent choices, not only because some essential oils can be expensive but also for my own satisfaction. I want to know not just how to do something but also why whatever I'm doing works—or not.

I didn't want to go through certification training to become an aromatherapist or spend hundreds of dollars. I simply wanted to understand how to choose oils for blending scents. As luck would have it, I discovered that an acquaintance of mine was working on certification in several natural healing methods, and aromatherapy was one of them. Best of all, she was willing to share some of her studies with me. Even though choosing oils for scent was a small part of her studies, it was enough to fill in the gaps in my knowledge. After spending some time with her, I felt like I was in heaven because I finally understood what I was doing with essential oils.

· · · · · · · ·

My interest in essential oils complements my interest in making herbal remedies, which is not surprising since the history of aromatic oils and of herbal medicine are intertwined. I grew up in a household where the first line of defense against illness or discomfort and the first aid rendered after injury usually came from the kitchen or my grandmother's garden. While commercial products eventually made their way into the family medicine cabinet, my mother often drifted back to remedies she knew as a child. Because of that, I became familiar with them too. The more I worked with essential oils, the more I found that they expanded and enhanced my herbal remedy repertoire.

Before going further, I must explain that I work with essential oils for my own purposes and not to provide treatment for others or sell products. While it may seem odd then that I have written this book, my purpose is to encourage others to explore the fascinating world of essential oils without feeling intimidated. That said, while I want to inspire people to be creative, I also urge readers to do so with safety in mind.

I also wanted to put together a book that covers a lot of ground. The word *Complete* in the title is not a reference to the number of essential oils that are profiled. Instead, it reflects a holistic approach where understanding carrier oils and other important ingredients in homemade preparations is equally important. Although recipe suggestions are provided throughout the book, the emphasis is on understanding the various types of remedies. Explanations and step-by-step instructions guide you through selecting, making, and using the different preparations and methods of application. It also helps you get the most from the essential oils you have on hand.

Part 1 of this book starts with a historical overview of essential oils. It explains what they are and how they differ from other aromatic products. Likewise, carrier oils are explained and explored. Safety precautions are also covered. Even though essential oils are natural products, they are powerful and need to be used carefully and wisely. I do not recommend the ingestion of essential oils, which should be done only under the direction of a healthcare professional.

Part 2 provides an in-depth explanation of how to blend oils for scent. It includes two fundamental methods for selecting essential oils: perfume note and scent group. This section also takes a fun look at making special birthday blends based on sun signs. While each essential oil profile includes suggestions on oils that blend well together, the beauty of scent is in the nose of the beholder. Follow the selection methods and your nose to create blends that are uniquely yours.

I have always thought that the term *aromatherapy* is a limited description because it seems to imply that the only use of essential oils is for scent. In fact, they can be used topically to fight infection, heal skin problems, soothe sore muscles, and ease joint pain. Part 3 explores the role of essential oils in herbal medicine and contains details on how to make healing remedies. It also includes a listing of ailments, which oils to use, and which methods work best to administer them.

Part 4 covers personal care and well-being, with information on how to make your own skin and hair care preparations. It also covers the classic aromatherapy use of scents for the emotions and how essential oils can be used to enhance spiritual practices. Related to well-being is the use of scent in conjunction with the energy of the chakras. We will also explore essential oils with candles to bring a little magic into our lives.

Part 5 brings us to yet another practical application of essential oils, which is their use in the home for cleaning, freshening, and pest control. Using essential oils with common household products, such as vinegar, helps eliminate the need for chemical cleaners. That said, while not all essential oils are appropriate for cleaning, all of them can be used in what I call *aromatic feng shui*. Details in chapter 15 take you step by step through a simple method for using essential oils with this ancient Chinese practice. Part 6 presents in-depth profiles of over sixty essential oils. Part 7 provides information on the carrier oils and other important ingredients commonly used in homemade preparations, including what type of water to use. Finally, the appendix contains measurement conversions and oil dilution charts, and the glossaries help support your exploration and learning.

There are a few well-known essential oils that are not included in this book. Rosewood (*Aniba rosaeodora*), also called *bois de rose*, is on the International Union for Conservation of Nature (IUCN) Red List of Endangered Species. This tree has been overexploited, and according to the IUCN, there are no significant signs of regeneration for the species. Spikenard (*Nardostachys jatamansi*) is also on the red list and is considered critically endangered. Indian sandalwood (*Santalum album*) is a scent that many of us adore, but unfortunately its popularity and overuse is causing its destruction. The IUCN considers sandalwood a vulnerable species, one step away from endangered. However, all is not lost, because the Australian government regulates the harvest of its species of sandalwood (*Santalum spicatum*) to ensure sustainability.

Occasionally, more than one essential oil can be obtained from a plant. For example, one type of oil comes from the roots of angelica and another from the seeds. Where it is important to make a distinction, I have noted them as angelica (root) or angelica (seed). Otherwise, just the word *angelica* refers to both oils. For oils where more than one species is represented, a similar distinction is made. For example, when a specific species of eucalyptus is referenced, it is noted as eucalyptus (blue) or eucalyptus (lemon). Just the word *eucalyptus* indicates that either oil can be used.

This book is intended to help you get the most from the essential oils you like and have on hand. While some recipes suggest certain oil combinations, the emphasis is on helping you create your own. If a recipe includes an oil that you do not have, check the quick guide of ailments and other tables throughout the book for oils that can be substituted.

You do not need a long list of ingredients to make an effective remedy. In fact, for centuries herbalists made "simples," remedies prepared with only one herb. Working with one herb or essential oil is a good way to get to know it and understand how it works for you.

The remedies in this book are geared to making small amounts so they are quick and easy to prepare. This also ensures that your preparations are fresh. Now let's step into the fascinating and life-enhancing world of essential oils.

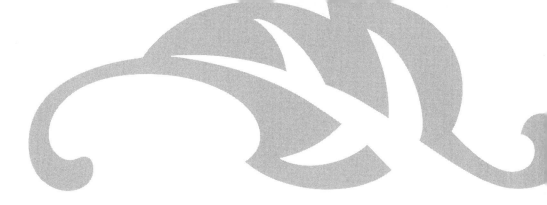

PART ONE

Background Information

In this section, we begin with a historical overview of essential oils and our fascination with scented oils. We will see how aromatic oils were used for medicinal and religious practices in many cultures throughout the ancient world. In addition, distilling aromatic plants into essential oils may be older than originally thought. During the twentieth century, chemicals were used extensively in manufacturing medicine and perfume; however, we will see how essential oils have made a comeback

From history, we will move into a little bit of science to learn what constitutes an essential oil, why plants produce them, and how these oils differ from other aromatic products on the market. We will learn about the various methods for obtaining essential oils and the by-products produced from them. Because a few products are often confused with essential oils, we will examine the other processes for producing different types of aromatic extracts.

Since essential oils are not used on their own, the refining methods for producing carrier oils are also detailed. After learning about these processes, you might change your mind about the oil you cook with. Marketing terms and red flags to watch out for when purchasing essential and carrier oils are also included.

While the common names of plants are easy to remember, they can be a source of confusion. Getting the correct essential oil is important, because even similar ones can have different properties and precautions. Although essential oils are natural alternatives to synthetic chemical-based products, they can be dangerous and harmful if used improperly. Without getting too technical, we will demystify their botanical names so you can be sure of getting the right oil. We will also cover safety precautions for ourselves, our families, and our pets.

· · · · · · · ·

CHAPTER I

The History of Essential Oils

The history of essential oils predates their manufacture and begins with the attraction that people have had with scented oils since ancient times. Aromatic plants steeped in oil were used as elements of religious and therapeutic practices in early cultures throughout the world. It was widely believed that scent provided a connection between the physical and spiritual worlds. Anointing with perfumes and fragrant oils was an almost universal practice that continues to this day. The word *perfume* comes from the Latin *per*, meaning "through," and *fume*, "smoke."[1]

Ancient Use of Scented Oils

Dating to the sixteenth century BCE, the Ebers Papyrus is the oldest written record on the use of medicinal plants in Egypt.[2] Along with the physical details of plants, it contains herbal recipes and information on perfumery and incense. Egyptian physicians often served as perfumers, producing medicinal oils that doubled as fragrance. Those who specialized in embalming the dead also used their expertise by creating mixtures to beautify the skin and protect it from the damaging harshness of the desert climate.

Always a valuable commodity, frankincense was regarded as the perfume of the gods. It was used in temple rites and as a base for personal perfume. Because aromatic oils were highly prized, the use of them remained in the province of the upper classes. These oils were often kept in exquisite bottles made of alabaster, jade, and other precious materials that were functional as well as beautiful. Some of these flasks retained scent until archaeologists opened them thousands of years after being sealed.

1. Groom, *The New Perfume Handbook*, 177.
2. Dobelis, ed., *Magic and Medicine of Plants*, 51.

The Babylonians also used aromatic plants and became a major supplier of plant material to neighboring countries. Cedarwood, cypress, myrtle, and pine were highly prized. The Assyrians were also fond of aromatics for religious rituals as well as personal use.

Some of the earliest writings from India, known as the *Vedas* (c. 1500 BCE), contain praises to the natural world, along with information about aromatics, including cinnamon, coriander, ginger, myrrh, sandalwood, and spikenard.[3] This information served as the backbone for Ayurvedic medicine, which is believed to be the oldest system of healing. Although the tenth-century Persian physician and philosopher Ibn Sina (980–1037), also known as Avicenna, is often credited with discovering the distillation process, archaeological evidence suggests that distilling aromatic plants into essential oils was achieved in India around 3000 BCE.[4]

The roots of Traditional Chinese Medicine began with a text called *The Yellow Emperor's Classic of Internal Medicine*, which included the use of aromatics. Phoenician merchants traded scented oils around the Mediterranean, bringing aromatic treasures from the Far East to Europe, most notably to the Greeks and Romans.

As the popularity of perfumes increased among the Greeks, the medicinal properties of herbs and oils became common knowledge. Unlike Egyptians, Greeks at all levels of society used aromatic oils. The ancient Romans carried on the Greek use of botanicals for medicinal and perfumery purposes. In addition, they scented their entire surroundings, from their bodies, clothes, and homes to public baths and fountains.

After the fall of the Roman Empire, the use of perfumery waned as Europe was plunged into the Dark Ages. To escape the upheaval, those who could afford it relocated to Constantinople (modern Istanbul, Turkey), and along with them went a storehouse of knowledge. As European civilization foundered, the works of Hippocrates and others were translated and widely distributed throughout the Middle East.

Medieval Times

Experimentation with plants continued and, as mentioned, Avicenna extracted essential oil, producing *otto* (or *attar*), the oil of flowers—in this case, rose. When European culture slowly recovered, the practice of perfumery spread from the Middle East to Spain, where it became exceedingly popular. After the Crusades, the perfumes of Arabia were in great demand throughout the Continent, and by the thirteenth century, a booming trade between the Middle East and Europe was reestablished.

The German physician Hieronymus Brunschwig (c. 1450–c. 1512) experimented with and wrote a comprehensive volume about the distillation process in which he mentioned juniper,

3. Chevallier, *The Encyclopedia of Medicinal Plants*, 34.
4. Başer and Buchbauer, eds., *Handbook of Essential Oils*, 6.

rosemary, and spike lavender essential oils. Intended mainly to create aromatic water, essential oil was considered a by-product. However, German naturalist and herbalist Adam Lonicer (1528–1586) viewed the process the other way around and placed more value on the essential oil than the aromatic water. Lonicer experimented with and wrote about sixty-one essential oils. He was instrumental in introducing their use into herbal medicine.[5]

By the middle of the sixteenth century, perfumery made a comeback throughout Europe and essential oil became popular for masking body odor. In France, fragrance was used as in ancient Rome: on the person, in the home, and in public fountains. Experimenting with local plants, Europeans began distilling lavender, rosemary, and sage.

Through the seventeenth and eighteenth centuries, pharmacists continued to study essential oils. The research of French chemists Antoine Lavoisier (1743–1794) and Jean-Baptiste Dumas (1800–1884) brought essential oils into wide use by the latter part of the nineteenth century. As chemists were able to isolate and study the components of essential oils, they also began to synthesize them in the laboratory.

The Modern Era

In the early twentieth century, the advancement of chemistry was overtaking the use of herbs and essential oils not only in medicines but in perfumes and cosmetics as well, because synthetic fragrance was cheaper and easier to produce. Ironically, it was a French chemist, René-Maurice Gattefossé (1881–1950), who was responsible for resurrecting the use of essential oils during the 1920s. After burning his hand in his laboratory, he grabbed the nearest bottle of liquid, which turned out to be lavender essential oil. Intrigued by the rapid healing that followed, he devoted the remainder of his career to studying essential oils and named his discovery *aromatherapy*.

Although chemicals were used extensively in manufacturing medicine and perfume during the twentieth century, the rise of the ecology movement spurred awareness of how our health depends on the health of the planet. Shifting attitudes ushered in an interest in herbal medicine, essential oils, and other natural healing methods and disciplines. As more of these "alternatives" make their way into mainstream use, we are finding that a mix of traditional and conventional medicine can give us the best of both worlds.

5. Ibid.

CHAPTER 2

Essential Oil Extraction Processes

Plants produce essential oils for various reasons such as aiding growth, attracting insects for pollination, and protecting against fungi or bacteria. Most plants produce essential oils in small quantities, but the plants commonly called *aromatics* create enough for us to harvest and enjoy. Essential oils are obtained from various parts of plants, and depending on the plant, it may produce separate oils from different parts. For example, angelica yields oil from both its roots and its seeds. Essential oil can be extracted from leaves, stems, and twigs; flowers and flower buds; citrus peel or the whole fruit; wood and bark; resin, oleoresin, and gum; roots, rhizomes, and bulbs; and seeds, kernels, and nuts.

Most of us have an idea of what an essential oil is, but the term is often mistakenly applied to a broad range of aromatic products from almost any natural source. There are two key aspects to essential oils. One is that they dissolve in alcohol or oil but not in water. The second is that they evaporate when exposed to air. Most essential oils are liquid, but some, such as rose oil, may become a semisolid depending on room temperature.

Distillation and Expression

The defining factor of what constitutes an essential oil is the method used to extract the oil from the plant material. Also called *volatile* oils, essential oils are obtained through the processes of distillation and expression. This differs from an aromatic extract, which is obtained through solvent extraction. The products created by solvent extraction contain both volatile and nonvolatile components. Let's take a closer look at these processes and the products produced from them.

The oldest and easiest method to obtain essential oil is called *expression*, or *cold pressing*. *Cold-pressed* may be a familiar term to those who enjoy cooking with olive oil. For essential oils, this extraction process works only with citrus fruit, because they hold a large amount of oil near the surface of their rinds. Depending on the plant, the whole fruit or just the peel is crushed and then the volatile oil is separated from the rest of the plant material by means of a centrifuge. This simple mechanical method does not require heat or chemicals. However, if the plants were not organically grown, there is a chance that the fruit was sprayed with pesticide, and trace amounts of it may remain in the oil.

The other process for extracting essential oil, called *distillation*, uses steam or water. During the distillation process, the volatile and soluble parts of a plant are separated, allowing the essential oil to be collected. Sometimes oils are distilled a second time to further purify them and rid them of any soluble material that may have been left behind the first time.

When steam is used in the process, it is pumped into the distillation container from underneath the plant material. Heat and pressure produced by the steam cause the plant material to break down and release its volatile oil. The oil is vaporized and transported with the steam through the still into a condenser unit, where it is cooled. The cooling process returns the oil and water to a liquid state. Depending on the density of the oil, it will either float to the top or sink to the bottom of the water. Either way, it is easily separated out. Different plants, as well as various parts of plants, require different amounts of time and temperatures for this process.

A method called *hydrodiffusion* is a form of distillation where the steam is forced into the vessel from above rather than below the plant material. The advantages are that it takes less steam and generally a shorter amount of time for this process. Some perfumers believe that hydrodiffusion produces a richer aroma than the standard steam distillation.

When water is used in the distillation process instead of steam, plant material is completely immersed in hot water. This process requires less pressure and slightly lower temperatures than steam distillation. Nevertheless, some plants, such as clary sage and lavender, tend to break down in this process. On the other hand, because some plants, such as neroli (orange blossom), are sensitive to high temperatures, water distillation works better with them.

After the essential oil is separated from the water in the distillation process, the water itself is an aromatic by-product called a *hydrosol*. Traditionally, these have been called *floral waters* (i.e., *rosewater*) and contain the water-soluble molecules of aromatic plants. Hydrosols are also called *hydroflorates* and *hydrolats*. The latter name comes from the Latin *latte* (familiar to coffee drinkers) and means "milk." It was so named because floral waters appear somewhat cloudy or milky just after they are separated from the essential oil. Although they are chemically different from their corresponding essential oils, the fragrance is similar. Because hydrosols are water-based substances, they do not mix well with oils. Also, hydrosols should not be used in place of flower essence remedies, as they are not prepared under the same conditions required for consumable products.

· · · · · · · ·

The term *flower essence* may cause some confusion because these products are not fragrant and they are not essential oils. They are simply an infusion of flowers in water, which is then mixed with a 50% brandy solution. Whereas the brandy acts as a preservative for flower essences, hydrosols can go bad.

The heat employed in steam and water distillation can cause changes to the plant material and the resulting oil. Sometimes this can be a good thing, but at other times, not so much. For example, heat converts the chemical matricin in German chamomile to chamazulene, which gives the oil its blue color. Medicinally, this is considered advantageous because the chamazulene makes the oil useful as an anti-inflammatory. On the other hand, jasmine flowers are so delicate that heat or water destroys their volatile oil.

Other Methods of Extraction

To avoid the negative effects that heat and water have on some plants, a solvent extraction process is used to obtain essential oil. Chemicals such as butane, hexane, ethanol, methanol, or petroleum ether are used in this process to rinse the volatile oil from the plant material. This rinsing produces a semisolid waxy product called a *concrete*, which, in addition to the volatile oil, contains the plant's waxes and fatty acids. In the case of jasmine, the concrete is 50% wax and 50% volatile oil. An advantage of a concrete is that it is more stable and concentrated than an essential oil.

Further rinsing with alcohol or ethanol and sometimes a freezing process can be used to remove the solvents and waxes. The result of this process is a substance called an *absolute*. While an absolute is usually a viscous liquid, it can also be a solid or semisolid. Absolutes are highly concentrated and have stronger, richer fragrances that are often more like the plant itself than the essential oil, which is advantageous for perfumery. The solvent extraction method produces a greater yield than distillation and is generally preferred for plants that have low quantities of oil. Absolutes and concretes are sometimes distilled to produce an essential oil. However, the basic problem with absolutes and concretes and the oils distilled from them is that they contain impurities: traces of the chemicals used to separate the oil from the plant material.

To avoid the problem of impurities, a method called *CO2 extraction*, sometimes called *supercritical CO2 extraction*, was developed. This process uses carbon dioxide in a liquid state at high pressure to dissolve plant material and release the oil. Afterward, when the pressure is reduced, the carbon dioxide returns to its gaseous state, leaving the oil behind and reportedly no chemical residue, as in the typical solvent extraction. However, like solvent extraction, CO2 extracts also contain plant fats, waxes, and resins.

There are two types of CO2 extraction products. One is created at lower pressure and is called a *select extract*, or *SE*. It is a liquid and does not contain as much of a plant's fat, waxes, and resins.

• • • • • • • •

The other type of CO2 extraction is called a *total extract*. It is thicker than the select extract and contains more of the nonsoluble plant material. According to Ingrid Martin, author and instructor of aromatherapy, lab tests revealed that there are "significant differences in chemical composition" between true essential oils and the CO2 products.[6]

Another substance created by the standard solvent extraction is called a *resinoid*. As the name implies, it comes from resinous plant material, which includes resins, balsams, oleoresins, and oleo-gum resins. (Refer to the glossary for information on these substances.) A resinoid can be in the form of a viscous liquid, a solid, or a semisolid. A further extraction process using alcohol produces a product called a *resin absolute*.

Another method of extraction is called *enfleurage*. This is rarely used today because it is extremely time-consuming and labor-intensive, thus making it very costly. This process is used to create an absolute from expensive flowers such as jasmine. Instead of extracting the essential oil with a chemical solvent, a fatty substance such as tallow or lard is used. This process involves coating a framed sheet of glass with the fat and then placing a layer of flowers in it. Another frame of glass is placed on top of the flowers, which in turn is coated with fat, on which a layer of flowers is placed, and so on.

Once a day, the whole array of glass frames is disassembled, the flowers picked out, and new ones placed in the same fat, and then everything is stacked again. This process goes on until the fat becomes saturated with volatile oil. The number of days it takes depends on the type of flower; jasmine takes about seventy days. On the final day when the flowers are removed, the fat is rinsed with alcohol to separate the oil from it. When the alcohol evaporates, an absolute is left. This type of absolute itself is sometimes called an *enfleurage*.

Another product is called *infused oil*. It is created through an easy, low-cost process of soaking plant material in vegetable oil to infuse it with a plant's aroma and chemistry. While infused oil has some medicinal value and is great for cooking, a very low amount of essential oil is released into the oil. (See more about infused oils in part 7.) Also called *maceration*, infusion is a very old method that was used by the ancient Egyptians. Infused oil has a well-earned place in herbal medicine and cooking, but keep in mind that this is not an essential oil, and it should not be priced or passed off as one.

Watch for Red Flags

There are a few things to watch for when purchasing essential oils. The first is synthetic oils. While these are lower in cost, they are also lower in quality because they are created chemically, usually with petroleum by-products instead of plant material. Although these oils may smell similar to the real thing, they do not carry the healing properties of essential oil. Another thing

6. Martin, *Aromatherapy for Massage Practitioners*, 13.

. . . .

to be aware of is dilution in carrier oil. A simple way to test for this is to put a drop of essential oil on a piece of paper. After it evaporates, there should be no trace left behind. An oily mark on the paper indicates the presence of a carrier oil.

Pricing is a red flag too. If a company's essential oils all cost about the same, it usually indicates that they are adulterated or synthetic oils. Some plants are simply more expensive than others, and this is reflected in the price of essential oils. The term *nature-identical* is another red flag that usually indicates an oil is synthetic or that a natural oil has been adulterated. In my mind, nature is nature, period. There is nothing "identical" to it. A final point to note is that essential oils come from plants and not animals. Musk, civet, and other oils from animals or birds should not be classified as essential oils.

Now that we know what to look for in essential oils, let's explore how carrier oils are produced.

CHAPTER 3

Carrier Oils

The reason for using carrier oils is that essential oils can cause irritation or other problems if applied directly to the body. Carrier oils are also called *base oils* or *fixed oils* because they serve as a base or fixed base and they do not evaporate when exposed to air, as essential oils do. Essential oils are very lipophilic, which means that they are readily absorbed by fatty oils and waxes. An example of this is the enfleurage method of essential oil extraction by laying flower petals in lard or tallow.

Because carrier oils are produced from the fatty portions of plants, they easily absorb essential oils, which become diluted as they are dispersed throughout the carrier oil. Most carrier oils are produced from seeds, kernels, or nuts. A few, such as avocado and olive, come from fruit. If you or anyone who will use your blends or remedies has a nut allergy, avoid using carrier oils produced from nuts.

Even though standard vegetable oils from the supermarket are sometimes recommended for use as carriers, we will explore why this is not such a good idea. Likewise, avoid the use of mineral or baby oil, because these are made from petroleum products.

Because carrier oils come from fatty plant matter, they can go rancid if not stored properly. Like essential oils, they should be kept in dark, airtight bottles, away from sun and artificial light. Storing them in the refrigerator can help keep them fresh and extend the shelf life. However, like anything else we keep in the fridge, they can eventually go bad, so if an oil does not look or smell right, throw it away.

Most carrier oils have a light scent that can be sweet, nutty, herbaceous, or spicy. These are not as strong as the aromatic oils and generally do not interfere with perfume blends. In some cases, you may find that the carrier oil's aroma can enhance the overall fragrance of a blend. Buy small quantities of carrier oil and experiment to see what works best with your creations.

· · · · · · · ·

Oil Refining Processes

At this point, you may be thinking that the standard vegetable oil from the supermarket doesn't have any smell. This is because chemical solvents are used to bleach and deodorize them and kill bacteria. While this extends the shelf life, it also means that we are putting chemicals into and onto our bodies.

Whether you are buying carrier oil or cooking oil, select one that is unrefined. If possible, buy organic oils. Refined oils are produced as cheaply as possible with the aid of solvents. Some are produced from genetically modified plants.

Refined food grade oils are produced to have no odor and very little to no color. For some reason, this has been considered a good thing. Some of the plant material harvested to make these oils is often stored for a year or more before being processed. When it is finally hauled out, the raw material is washed with chemicals to remove any mold that may have grown on it while in storage.

This initial wash down is followed by a solvent extraction process, which separates the oil from the plant solids. Next comes the distillation process to remove the chemicals used in the wash down. The resulting goop, called *crude oil*, is then filtered. While you and I might think of the nice clean filters we use in coffee machines, this filtration process involves heating the oil and adding sodium hydroxide (also known as lye) or sodium carbonate (a sodium salt of carbonic acid) to neutralize it. But wait, there's more. Fuller's earth (aluminum silicate) or a clay-based earth is used to remove as much color as possible. These earths are very fine-grained and highly absorbent of impurities and dirt. They also remove the molecules that create the oil's color.

The cycle continues. After one process adds something to the oil, it is followed by another process to remove whatever was put in. The oil is filtered again to remove the earths. It is then put through a steam vacuum at high temperatures to deodorize it. After wringing most of the nutrients out of it, the oil is subjected to one last process called *winterizing*, which keeps it from turning cloudy at lower temperatures. Unrefined oils may appear cloudy when stored in the fridge, but this does not change their chemical compositions or nutritional and healing properties. I prefer the clouds and shorter shelf life for my oils.

Marketing Terms

You may encounter some carrier oils called *partially refined*. This means that the oil was subjected to some of the processes described above, which most often includes bleaching, deodorizing, and winterizing. However, some of the other processes may have been employed as well. Partial refining is used to stabilize oils that normally have a short shelf life. It also neutralizes oils that have a darker color or stronger smell.

Some other terms encountered when buying oils include the word *pure*, which simply means that it was not mixed with any other type of oil. The word *natural* on the label means that it was not diluted with a synthetic oil, and the word *organic* indicates that the plants were grown according to certain standards.

An unrefined oil may be labeled *cold pressed*, which means that it was not subjected to high temperatures. As we learned in the previous chapter about essential oil extraction methods, cold-pressing is a mechanical process that does not apply heat. However, some heat is generated from the press mechanism, but it normally stays under 60–80°F (approximately 15–26°C). A similar method called *expeller pressed* employs hydraulic presses. While external heat is not applied in this method either, friction generated by this type of press can raise the heat level up to 200°F (approximately 93°C). Using a hydraulic press is less costly, making the oil a little more economical. In my research, sources have indicated that this amount of heat does not harm the oil.

Plant material is usually put through a press more than once to squeeze out as much oil as possible. Oil that is extracted from the first pressing is called *virgin*. After the final pressing, the oil is put through cotton cloth filters and then paper filters to remove any bits of plant material. Finally, it's ready for bottling.

In the next chapter, we will learn why scientific names are important and the safety precautions we should keep in mind when choosing and using essential oils.

CHAPTER 4

❧

The Importance of Scientific Names and Safety Guidelines

While the common names of plants are easy to remember, they can be a source of confusion because a plant may be known by multiple names or two plants can share a common name. For example, the kitchen herb bay (*Laurus nobilis*) shares its common name with West Indian bay (*Pimenta racemosa*). Essential oils from both plants are available and are sometimes simply called *bay*. The problem is that these oils have different medicinal uses and precautions. For this reason, it is important to know the botanical names (genus and species) when purchasing essential and carrier oils to be sure of getting the right ones.

Genus and species are part of a complex naming structure devised by Swedish naturalist Carl Linnaeus (1707–1778), whose work became the foundation for the International Code of Botanical Nomenclature (which was changed to the International Code of Nomenclature for Algae, Fungi, and Plants in 2011). Over time, as new knowledge about plants emerged, their names were changed to reflect new data.

This is one reason why we find synonyms in botanical names. The antiquated names are not completely dropped because they aid in identification. For example, marjoram is usually noted as *Origanum majorana*, syn. *Majorana hortensis*. Other reasons for synonyms are scientific disagreement and sometimes pride.

Most names are in Latin because during Linnaeus's time it was a common language for people engaged in scientific research. The first word in the botanical name is the plant's genus, which is often a proper noun and is always capitalized. The second word, the species name, is an adjective that usually provides something descriptive about the plant. For example, the genus for coriander, *Coriandrum*, is the Latin name for the plant, which was derived from the Greek *koriannon*. The

· · · · · · · ·

species name, *sativum*, is also Latin and means "cultivated."[7] Occasionally, you may see a third word preceded by "var.", indicating that the plant is a variety of that species. For example, the botanical names for bergamot are *Citrus bergamia* syn. *C. aurantium* var. *bergamia*.

You may also see a multiplication sign (×) in a name, which indicates that the plant is a hybrid—a cross between two plants. For example, peppermint, *Mentha × piperita*, is a naturally occurring hybrid between spearmint (*Mentha spicata*) and water mint (*Mentha aquatica*). A letter or an abbreviation sometimes follows a botanical name, identifying the person who named the plant. For example, "F. Muell." is the abbreviation for Ferdinand von Mueller (1825–1896), a German-Australian botanist. The letter "L." at the end of a botanical name means that Linnaeus himself bestowed it.

While it is not necessary to memorize botanical names, it is a good idea to jot them down to have handy while shopping for essential oils. As mentioned, getting the correct oil is important because even similar ones can have different properties and precautions.

Safety First

My purpose for writing this book is to encourage others to explore, have fun, and reap the benefits of essential oils without feeling intimidated. However, working with them must be done with knowledge and common sense. Although essential oils are natural alternatives to synthetic chemical-based products, they must be used with safety in mind.

Essential oils, like plants, may be dangerous and harmful if used improperly, which is why it is important to store them out of reach of children. Pregnant and breastfeeding women and anyone with a medical condition should take extra care. Read and heed warning information. In general, avoid rubbing your eyes or handling a contact lens if you have oil on your fingers, as some oils may irritate eyes and damage contact lenses. If you get essential oil in your eye, flush it with cold milk to dilute the oil. The fatty lipids in milk act the same as carrier oils. Because essential oils are not water-soluble, water would only spread the oil around and not help to remove it. Also, avoid getting oil vapors in your eyes, as they can cause irritation too.

Essential oils should not be taken internally without the advice of a physician or trained healthcare provider. When using topical remedies to treat minor problems, it is important to work with your doctor if a problem becomes prolonged or escalates.

As mentioned, essential oils must be diluted before being used on the body; lavender is the only exception. While sandalwood and ylang-ylang are considered very gentle and are often used for perfume, it is important to do a patch test first and read any warning information before doing so.

To do a patch test, put a couple of drops of essential oil on your wrist, then cover it loosely with an adhesive bandage. After a couple of hours, remove the bandage and check for any red-

---

7. Cumo, ed., *Encyclopedia of Cultivated Plants*, 436.

• • • • • • • •

ness or signs of irritation. If these occur, rinse the area with cold milk. You may try the test again at another time or on the other wrist with the essential oil diluted in a carrier oil. If you have sensitive skin, it is advisable to always do a patch test with diluted oils.

While there are exceptions and each person may react differently to an oil, it is best to err on the side of caution. Read the manufacturer's label, and when in doubt, don't use it. People with epilepsy or other seizure disorders and those with high blood pressure should consult their doctors before using essential oils. You may also want to consult your pediatrician before using essential oils on children. In general, small amounts of essential oils are used on children and older adults. The following table lists the general warnings and safety issues for the essential oils included in this book. Check the individual profiles in part 6 for further precautions.

Table 4.1 Safety Guidelines for Essential Oils

Children
Avoid the use of these oils on children, especially under the age of six: anise seed, black pepper, cajeput, cardamom, citronella, eucalyptus (blue), fennel, geranium, lemongrass, peppermint (children under twelve), pine, ravintsara, rosemary.

Dermal Irritation
These oils may cause irritation to the skin, especially if used in high concentrations: anise seed, basil, bay laurel, black pepper, cajeput, caraway seed, cedarwood, chamomile, cinnamon leaf, citronella, clove bud, elemi, eucalyptus, fir needle, ginger, grapefruit, helichrysum, juniper berry, lemon, lemon balm, lemongrass, orange, peppermint, pine, ravintsara, spearmint, rosemary, sandalwood.

Epilepsy or Seizure Disorders
These oils should be avoided: fennel, hyssop, rosemary.

High Blood Pressure
Avoid these oils: hyssop, peppermint, pine, rosemary, thyme.

Homeopathy
These oils should not be used when undergoing homeopathic treatment: black pepper, eucalyptus, peppermint, spearmint.

Medications
Check the use of these oils with certain medications: bay laurel, clary sage, grapefruit, lavender.

Moderation
These oils should be used in moderation: anise seed, basil, bay laurel, black pepper, cinnamon leaf, clove bud, coriander, eucalyptus, fennel, hyssop, juniper berry, marjoram, peppermint, sage, ylang-ylang.

Table 4.1 Safety Guidelines for Essential Oils (*continued*)

Phototoxic

These oils may cause a rash or dark pigmentation on skin exposed to sunlight/UV light within twelve to eighteen hours after application: angelica (root), bergamot, ginger, grapefruit, lemon, lime, mandarin, orange.

Pregnancy

These oils should be avoided during pregnancy: angelica, anise seed, basil, bay laurel, black pepper, carrot seed, cedarwood (Atlas), cinnamon leaf, citronella, clary sage, clove bud, coriander, cypress, fennel, frankincense, geranium, hyssop, juniper berry, lemongrass, marjoram, myrrh, peppermint, pine, ravintsara, rose, rosemary, sage, thyme.
Abortifacient: cedarwood (Virginia)

Sensitization

These oils may sensitize the skin: bay laurel, fennel, geranium, ginger, hyssop, lemon, lemon balm, palmarosa, spearmint, tea tree.

Essential Oils and Pets

Just as we need to take precautions when using essential oils on our own bodies, it is even more important with pets, as they cannot explain what they are experiencing. While some essential oils are used for bathing dogs or calming their nerves, it is important to check with your veterinarian first. Just as the dilution ratio for humans differs from adult to child, it also varies according to a dog's size and whether it is a puppy. The age and condition of the dog should also be taken into consideration. In addition, not all essential oils that are safe for humans are safe for dogs. It is beyond the scope of this book to offer in-depth information, and I urge readers to research the issue before using essential oils with your pets.

When using essential oils on yourself, be sure they are fully absorbed before touching your pets. This is particularly important with cats and small animals. Cats are especially sensitive to odors, and special care must be taken when using essential oils in your home because they may be toxic to your feline. When using a diffuser or vaporizer, be sure your cat can easily move to another room. If you use essential oils for cleaning, avoid using them around the litter box or food bowls. Be sure that areas where you use essential oils for cleaning are thoroughly rinsed or vacuumed. Essential oils should never be used on a cat, because they will ingest them while cleaning themselves.

Also take precautions when using essential oils if you have small animals such as hamsters, guinea pigs, or rabbits. Do not diffuse essential oils in a room with fish or birds. As mentioned, check with your veterinarian, and do some research beyond a browse on the internet. With a little effort, you can enjoy the use of essential oils and keep your pets safe.

· · · · · · · ·

The Shelf Life of Essential Oils

Once you have purchased your essential oils, store them in a cool, dark, and dry environment. Avoid keeping them in the bathroom or kitchen, as the humidity and fluctuating temperatures of these rooms may damage the oils. Some experts recommend storing them in the fridge, especially if you live in a warm climate. If you store them this way, keep the bottles wrapped in plastic storage wrap or containers to avoid affecting the taste of food in the fridge.

Careful storage is important because exposure to heat, sunlight, moisture, and air causes degradation of essential oils. They become less potent, therapeutically and aromatically. In addition, oxidization causes a chemical change in the oils, which can pose hazards. Signs to watch for are cloudiness, thickening of the oil, or a change in its aroma. The best clue is a change in the aroma, because essential oils stored in the fridge tend to thicken a little and citrus oils become slightly cloudy when cool. A reducer cap helps prevent excess air from getting in the bottle. It also makes it easier to dispense thinner oils. Consider moving oils to progressively smaller bottles as you use them to help reduce the amount of air in the bottle during storage.

Because there are so many variables, including the quality of the oil and how it was handled prior to purchase, it is difficult to provide anything but an approximate shelf life. The following table gives a rough guideline.

Table 4.2 Rough Guide to the Shelf Life of Essential Oils

9 to 12 Months
Angelica, cypress, fir needle, pine, most oils from citrus peel (except bergamot), grapefruit, lemon, lime, mandarin, orange
12 to 18 Months
Cajeput, frankincense, lemongrass, niaouli, tea tree
2 to 3 Years
Most oils that include bergamot, cedarwood (Virginia)   Lasting slightly longer: black pepper, carrot seed, cinnamon leaf, clove bud, eucalyptus, helichrysum, lavender, peppermint, ravintsara
4 to 6 Years
Cedarwood (Atlas), myrrh, patchouli, sandalwood, vetiver

Moving on to part 2, we will learn how to choose and blend essential oils to create personalized scents that can be used as perfumes or to add interest to personal care products.

· · · · · · · ·

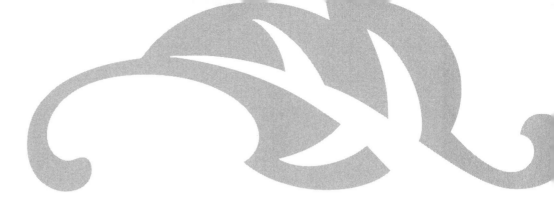

PART TWO

How to Choose and Blend Oils for Scent

This section provides information on two fundamental methods for selecting essentials oils for scent. Called *perfume note*, this popular method started with the nineteenth-century concept of equating scents with musical notes. Classifying smells according to musical scales was complex and cumbersome, but simplifying it to three notes made it manageable and easy to use. We will examine what constitutes each of the three notes, and because all oils do not fit neatly into one of the three categories, we will include the sliding scale of in-between notes.

The other method for choosing oils is by scent group, also called *fragrance groups* or *fragrance families*. There have been various methods for grouping scent, some more complicated than others. From the overly complex to the questionable, we will look at several interesting ways that odors have been classified. The method detailed in this section uses a simple set of six categories that provide three ways of selecting oils. Because scents are subjective, the methods for selecting essential oils provide a starting point for exploration. Let your nose be the ultimate guide.

In addition to the two fundamental methods for selecting scents, I have included a birthday blend. This is a unique and fun way to choose oils based on your zodiac sign. In addition to birthstones, plants and their essential oils have become associated with the zodiac constellations. With this method, we can create special blends for ourselves and make personalized gifts for others.

The final chapter in this section provides a step-by-step explanation of the blending process. Recipes for making liquid and solid perfumes are also included. Of course, a personal perfume blend can also be used to make bath bombs, shower melts, and other beauty products that are detailed in subsequent parts of this book.

. . . .

CHAPTER 5

꩜

Choosing Essential Oils by Perfume Note

One of the most popular methods for blending scents is by perfume note. This concept began with British analytical chemist and perfumer G. W. Septimus Piesse (1820–1882), who devised a method of classifying scents according to musical scales. As he explained in his book *The Art of Perfumery*, the method was based on his belief in the brain's link between sound and smell. According to Piesse, assigning fragrances to certain notes allowed the perfumer to create harmonious scents. For example, a C chord would result with a blend of sandalwood, geranium, acacia, neroli, and camphor. Piesse's son Charles is sometimes credited with devising this system, because as editor of the book, he removed his father's name from editions published after his death.

The Three-Note Scale

Piesse's system was complex, and the concept was not widely used until William Arthur Poucher (1891–1988) simplified it into three notes. Research chemist and chief perfumer at Yardley of London, Poucher began to classify scents based on their rates of volatility. His book *Perfumes Cosmetics and Soaps* has been in print since 1923 and is still a classic reference in the field of cosmetics. In his method, essential oils are assigned to one of three notes based on their dominant characteristic and rate of evaporation. The notes are usually called *top*, *middle*, and *base*.

The top note is also called the *head note* or *peak note*. It is the component that is first detected and is usually the strongest, but it has the most rapid evaporation rate, lasting only ten minutes to several hours. While the top note leads the way, it then gives way for the other components of a scent to take over. The middle note is also called the *heart note* or *modifier*. It is usually detectable ten

· · · · · · · ·

to forty-five minutes after the perfume is applied and can last for several hours to several days. The base note is also called the *body note* or *fixative*. Its purpose is to slow the rate of evaporation of the top note and to act as an anchor to hold the fragrance together. A base note scent can last for several days to over a week. Working together, the top note introduces the scent and the middle and base notes create the core of it. Mixing an oil from each of the three notes creates a well-rounded blend that unfolds over time.

Blending by Perfume Note

Although the theory is to use three notes, not all oils fit neatly into one category of top, middle, or base. Some oils are complex in that they can function as more than one note. Angelica seed oil is an example, and although it is often classified as a top note, it is in between the top and the middle. In addition to functioning as either note, an oil that is in between creates a bridge that smooths the separate notes in a blend.

In-between oils can serve as either note, depending on the other oils in a blend. For example, in a blend with neroli (middle), cedarwood (middle to base), and amyris (base), neroli serves as the top note and amyris as the base. A blend using peppermint (top), lavender (middle to top), and juniper berry (middle) shifts the scale upward but still maintains a three-note spread. Don't be afraid to experiment with note ranges. Have fun and explore.

As mentioned in the introduction, I have included details to distinguish between the species of plants where details differ. For example, German and Roman chamomile have different perfume notes. The same goes for angelica seed and root oils and a few others. In the case of eucalyptus, where both species have the same note, the single entry of *eucalyptus* applies to both.

Table 5.1 Perfume Notes of Essential Oils

Top	Middle to Top	Middle	Middle to Base	Base
Anise seed	Angelica (seed)	Caraway seed	Angelica (root)	Amyris
Bergamot	Basil	Cardamom	Black pepper	Frankincense
Fennel	Bay laurel	Carrot seed	Cedarwood	Myrrh
Lemon	Cajeput	Chamomile (Roman)	Chamomile (German)	Patchouli
Lime	Citronella	Cinnamon leaf	Clary sage	Sandalwood
Mandarin	Eucalyptus	Clove bud	Cypress	Vetiver
Peppermint	Grapefruit	Coriander	Ginger	
Ravintsara	Hyssop	Elemi	Helichrysum	
Rose	Lavender	Fir needle	Ylang-ylang	
Spearmint	Lemongrass	Geranium		
	Orange	Juniper berry		
	Petitgrain	Lemon balm		
	Pine	Manuka		
	Rosemary	Marjoram		
	Tea tree	Neroli		
	Thyme	Niaouli		
		Palmarosa		
		Sage		

When you begin mixing with this method, it is best to keep it simple by using three oils in a blend. This way, you will learn how each oil functions as its intended note and be better positioned to combine multiple oils of the same note in more complex blends.

The simple rule of thumb for blending by perfume note is to start with a 3:2:1 ratio—three drops of the top note, two drops of the middle note, and one drop of the base note. Even though the top note may be strong, it is more fleeting and can work in a higher amount. Once you have one drop of all three notes, add one drop of your middle note and then one of your top note. If all seems well, add one more of your top note.

Occasionally, you may find that a reverse formula is more to your liking, especially if you want to emphasize the lower note. Follow your nose and proceed slowly when adding drops as you develop your blend. Follow the procedure as detailed in chapter 7 for assessing and allowing a blend to mature. Some individual oils become deeper and richer over time, which will further enhance the development of a blend. These oils include frankincense, patchouli, and rose.

As with all blending methods, this is a starting point. After creating a couple of blends with three oils, you may want to experiment by doubling the number of oils for each note. Oils that seem to take over a blend can be tempered with others such as black pepper, lemon, or geranium to create more of a balance. You will also find that an emphasis on base notes can create a more spicy or earthy blend. While lavender and sandalwood are a wonderful and traditional combination, this mix can be jazzed up by adding a lemon top note. In addition, lavender or sandalwood can be used to enhance and bring out the beauty of other oils. Rosemary or marjoram can help smooth a blend.

In the next chapter, we will learn how to use scent groups for choosing essential oils and how to create a birthday blend based on your zodiac sign.

CHAPTER 6

Choosing Essential Oils by Scent Group and Sun Sign

Scents have been classified in several ways, some more complex than others. Carl Linnaeus revolutionized and standardized the classification of plants according to their physical structure and development, but he didn't stop there and went on to categorize their odors as well. However, his focus was on their medicinal value. Though not very inspirational for blending scents, he classified odors as *foul, fragrant, garlicky, goaty, musky, nauseating,* and *spicy.*

In 1916, German psychologist Hans Henning (1885–1946) called his six-odor system the *smell prism,* and in 1927, American chemical engineer Ernest Crocker (1888–1964) equated what he called the *odor square* with what he believed were four types of olfactory nerves.[8] Coming from a totally different viewpoint and with a different purpose, Eugene Rimmel (1820–1887), eminent perfumer of London and Paris, laid out his eighteen classifications of scents in *The Book of Perfumes.*

Perfume Categories

Today, perfume categories vary widely and sometimes require explanation. For example, the category called *green* generally includes herbs, mints, and pine; *oriental* includes heady spices and some resinous scents; *chypre* (French for "cypress") includes woodsy/mossy scents; and *fougère* (French for "fern") includes lighter herb or fern-like scents. Three of the more recent perfume

---

8. Stokes, Matthen, and Biggs, eds., *Perception and Its Modalities,* 226.

categories are called *fruity*, *gourmand* (an edible food smell), and *aquatic*, which accommodates synthetic fragrances.[9]

In addition to the square and the prism, the circle has also been employed to classify scents. The modern fragrance wheel developed by perfume aficionado Michael Edwards in the early 1980s has the category *fougère* at the hub, with the four categories of *floral*, *fresh*, *oriental*, and *woody* around the outside. The four latter categories are each divided into three or four subgroups.

As you may have guessed by now, scents are subjective. However, through my studies I found a method for categorizing scents that offers a simple, straightforward blending guide. The set of six scent groups recommended by aromatherapist, author, and lecturer Julia Lawless are illustrated in figure 6.1.[10]

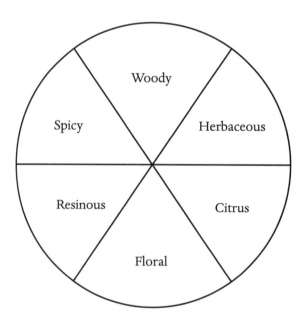

Figure 6.1 The Scent Group Wheel Provides Simple Guidance for Blending Perfumes

The groups consist of *woody* (woodsy, earthy), *herbaceous*, *citrus*, *floral*, *resinous*, and *spicy*. These groups describe something about the plants within the categories. Like Michael Edwards's groups, this set works well as a wheel because it shows their interrelationships and the dynamic nature of this blending method.

9. Groom, *The New Perfume Handbook*, 262.

10. Lawless, *The Illustrated Encyclopedia of Essential Oils*, 44.

Three Ways to Blend by Scent Group

There are three ways to use the scent groups for choosing oils. The first is what I call *single group* blending, because all the oils are selected from one scent group. It works because the members within each group tend to have similar chemical compositions and go well with one another. As a result, most of the floral scents blend well together, as do the spices, citrus, and other groupings. To help you, table 6.1 (later in this chapter) contains a listing of essential oils by scent group.

Once you have selected your oils, follow the steps laid out in chapter 7 to create your aromatic treasure. This will be the same for all the scent-blending methods, as the actual steps for mixing and assessing blends remain the same; it is the planning and selecting of oils that differs. When you purchase a new essential oil, you may want to label it with the name of its scent group, which will make it easier when planning new blends.

The second way of using scent groups is *good neighbor* blending. As this name implies, each group mixes well with members from its neighboring groups. The woody oils go well with the spicy and herbaceous oils, the citrus with herbaceous and floral oils, and so on. All around the circle, each group complements its neighbors on either side.

When blending this way, select your oils from two groups. For example, choose oils from the woody and spicy groups or the woody and herbaceous groups. That said, remember that these are simple guidelines. Once you are familiar with your oils and you feel that combining certain spicy, woody, and herbaceous oils would create a good blend, go for it.

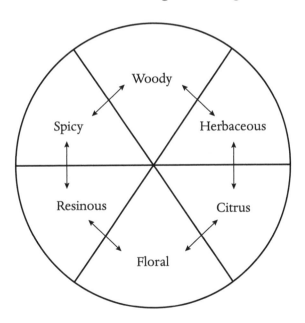

Figure 6.2 Each Scent Group Complements Its Neighbors

The third way of using scent groups is *opposite group* blending. As you can see in figure 6.3, these pairings are not completely straightforward. The woody and floral groups and the spicy and citrus groups are directly opposite each other on the circle, and these combinations work nicely. Although the herbaceous and resinous groups are opposites and some of their members go nicely together, this pairing of groups does not always work as well as the others. However, even though they are not opposites, the spicy and floral groups tend to work well together. Using one of your three oils from an opposite group adds interest to a blend and opens the door to a wide range of possibilities.

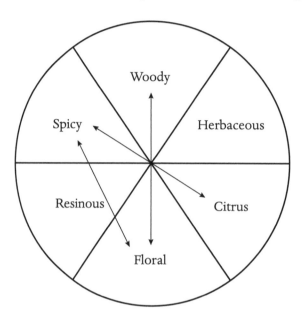

Figure 6.3 Scents from Opposite Groups Can Blend Well

Table 6.1 Essential Oils and Their Scent Groups

Woody	Amyris, cajeput, cedarwood, cypress, eucalyptus (blue), fir needle, juniper berry, patchouli, pine, ravintsara, sandalwood, vetiver
Herbaceous	Angelica, basil, carrot seed, chamomile, citronella, clary sage, helichrysum, hyssop, manuka, marjoram, niaouli, peppermint, rosemary, sage, spearmint, tea tree, thyme
Citrus	Bergamot, eucalyptus (lemon), grapefruit, lemon, lemon balm, lemongrass, lime, mandarin, orange
Floral	Geranium, lavender, neroli, palmarosa, rose, ylang-ylang
Resinous	Frankincense, myrrh
Spicy	Anise seed, bay laurel, black pepper, caraway seed, cardamom, cinnamon leaf, clove bud, coriander, elemi, fennel, ginger, petitgrain

Birthday Perfume Blends

Since ancient times, the constellations were believed to have an influence on people and provide omens or signs. During the Middle Ages, astrology was divided between the two applications of divination and medicine. The famed English herbalist Nicholas Culpeper (1616–1654) wrote several books on astrology and integrated this knowledge into his herbal practice. In addition to crystals (birthstones), plants and their essential oils have become associated with the zodiac signs.

Creating a birthday blend for someone makes a nice personalized gift. Table 6.2 contains a list of essential oils according to their associated sun signs. (The date ranges for the signs are approximate.) Some oils are associated with more than one sign. You may want to incorporate ideas from the perfume note and scent group methods for choosing your oils, or follow your nose and experiment.

Table 6.2 Essential Oils and Their Sun Signs

Capricorn (December 22 to January 19)
Cinnamon leaf, cypress, eucalyptus, manuka, myrrh, patchouli, pine, tea tree, vetiver
Aquarius (January 20 to February 18)
Anise seed, clary sage, cypress, frankincense, lavender, lemon, mandarin, myrrh, patchouli, peppermint, pine, rosemary, sage, sandalwood
Pisces (February 19 to March 20)
Anise seed, bay laurel, cardamom, clove bud, cypress, elemi, eucalyptus, lavender, lemon, manuka, myrrh, palmarosa, pine, sage, sandalwood, tea tree, ylang-ylang
Aries (March 21 to April 19)
Angelica, basil, black pepper, cardamom, cedarwood, cinnamon leaf, clove bud, coriander, fennel, fir needle, frankincense, geranium, ginger, juniper berry, marjoram, neroli, peppermint, petitgrain, pine, rosemary, thyme
Taurus (April 20 to May 20)
Cardamom, cedarwood, citronella, cypress, eucalyptus, helichrysum, patchouli, ravintsara, rose, sage, thyme, vetiver, ylang-ylang
Gemini (May 21 to June 21)
Anise seed, bay laurel, bergamot, caraway seed, fennel, grapefruit, helichrysum, lavender, lemon, lemongrass, marjoram, peppermint, ravintsara, spearmint, thyme
Cancer (June 22 to July 22)
Cardamom, chamomile, eucalyptus, geranium, hyssop, lemon, lemon balm, myrrh, palmarosa, pine, rose, sandalwood

· · · · · · ·

Table 6.2 Essential Oils and Their Sun Signs (*continued*)

Leo (July 23 to August 22)
Angelica, anise seed, basil, bay laurel, chamomile, cinnamon leaf, clove bud, frankincense, ginger, juniper berry, lavender, lime, neroli, niaouli, orange, petitgrain, rosemary, sandalwood
Virgo (August 23 to September 22)
Bergamot, carrot seed, cypress, fennel, grapefruit, lavender, marjoram, niaouli, patchouli, peppermint, rosemary, sandalwood
Libra (September 23 to October 23)
Amyris, clary sage, marjoram, ravintsara, rose, spearmint, thyme, vetiver
Scorpio (October 24 to November 21)
Basil, clary sage, clove bud, ginger, myrrh, niaouli, patchouli, pine, ravintsara
Sagittarius (November 22 to December 21)
Anise seed, cajeput, cedarwood, clove bud, frankincense, ginger, hyssop, juniper berry, manuka, orange, rose, rosemary, sage, tea tree

Now that we have learned several methods for choosing essential oils, we will go step by step through the process of blending and evaluating scents.

CHAPTER 7

Perfume Blending Basics

While mixing essential oils may seem like a no-brainer, there are a few steps that will help you get the most from your blending experience and add to your skills. The equipment needed for blending is minimal:

- Small bottles with screw-on caps for blending and storing essential oils and for mixing with carrier oils. You may want to have several sizes on hand.
- Small droppers to transfer essential and carrier oils into blending bottles.
- A medicine dropper with a teaspoon or milliliter gauge for measuring carrier oil. This is optional but a nice convenience.
- Small adhesive labels.
- A notebook and pen.
- Cotton swabs or perfume blotter strips/scent-testing strips. These are optional but a nice convenience.

All bottles used for essential oils should be a dark color and made of glass. A dark bottle prevents oil degradation caused by light. Most bottles on the market are usually amber or cobalt blue and come in a range of sizes. Never use plastic, because the bottle's chemical composition can interact with essential oil. The 2 and 5 milliliter bottles are good for blending essential oils, and the 15 and 30 milliliter sizes work well for combining them with carrier oil.

Have a separate dropper for each essential oil when transferring them to the blending bottle to avoid even a minor mixing of oils. Make sure that the bottles and droppers are clean and dry.

Many essential oil bottles have reducer caps, which help prevent excess air from getting inside and increasing the rate of oxidation. However, depending on the oil, you may want to remove the reducer cap. While the cap makes it easier to dispense thinner oils that sometimes pour out too quickly, it can be more difficult with thicker oils such as amyris, patchouli, and sandalwood.

You may want to do a drop test if you are using oils that vary in thickness. Put one drop of each oil that you are working with on a plate to compare sizes. Most of the thin oils will be about the same size, but a drop of a thicker oil will be noticeably larger. This is a point to remember when blending for scent or making remedies so you can keep the amounts in proportion.

It is best to work on a surface that is washable, because essential oils can damage varnish, paint, and plastic surfaces. It's also a good idea to put down a layer of paper towels on your work surface to catch any stray drops.

Ready, Set, Blend

For your first blend, start with three oils so it will be simple but interesting. In fact, more is not always better, and some lovely fragrances can be created using just two oils. The first step is to get familiar with the individual scents. Open one bottle of essential oil, then dip a cotton swab or blotter strip into the oil and gently waft it back and forth under your nose.

Close your eyes for a moment and allow the scent to speak to you. Does it evoke any sensation, emotion, or image? Take notes on your impressions as well as the oil's initial strength. Strength is usually classified as light, mild, medium, strong, or very strong. This information will be useful when planning future blends.

After sampling an oil's scent, set the swab or blotter strip aside. You may also want to walk into another room to clear your nose of the fragrance before moving on to the next oil. Although I have not tried it, I have heard that wafting fresh coffee grounds under the nose can clear the olfactory sense. When you are ready, repeat the sampling process for the other oils in your blend.

The last step before mixing the oils is to take all three swabs or blotter strips and waft them together under your nose. While this can provide a sneak preview of the blend, you will know how well it works only after the oils are mixed and have had time to settle and mature.

Using separate droppers, put one drop of each essential oil, beginning with the base note, into the blending bottle. As you'll recall, the base oils are also called a *fixative* because they hold a scent together.

While Agent 007 may have preferred his martini shaken, not stirred, for mixing oils we want to swirl, not shake. After a few swirls, waft the bottle near your nose to preview the blend. Keep in mind the initial intensity of each oil. If one oil is a lot stronger than the other two, add a drop more of the others. If the oils are different strengths, adjust the amounts accordingly, but add only one drop at a time and walk away for a moment before sampling the fragrance again. Be sure to take notes on how many drops of each oil you add.

At this point, the blend is in its infancy, but don't be afraid to make corrections. If your nose tells you that a drop more of an oil would be better, try it. This is the way to learn and hone your skills. However, if the mix seems like it's almost right or if you're not sure about it, refrain from adding more. Instead, put the lid on the bottle, wash the droppers, and let the blend settle for a couple of hours before taking another whiff. After you do so, take notes about any differences you may detect. Unless you are unhappy with the blend at this point, don't tinker with it.

Give the blend a couple of days before you do another smell test. Again, refrain from adjusting it during this time period; let the oils work their magic. Next comes the hard part of waiting at least a week to give the blend time to mature. It takes time for the chemistry of the oils to change and develop as some molecules will break up and form new ones with the other oils. You may be surprised to find that something you thought needed a tweak has turned into an aromatic jewel.

Taking notes at each step is important, because when you find the right blend, you can easily duplicate it and increase the amount. And on occasion (I speak from experience), you may not want to repeat it. It happens and that's how we learn, although understanding the oil selection methods increases your chances of producing a winner.

Label the bottle with the date and give your blend a name or simply list the ingredients. Keep the bottle tightly closed in a cool place away from light. Also, be sure to keep it out of reach of children.

Making Your Own Perfume

After your aromatic creation has had a week or so to mature, it can be added to a carrier oil and used. As mentioned, carrier oils are important because essential oils should never be used full strength on the skin due to potential irritation.

Be sure to use separate droppers for the carrier oil and the essential oils. As noted in the list of equipment, you might want to purchase a dropper with a milliliter or teaspoon gauge to make it easier to measure the carrier oil. These can be found in most pharmacies. Also, for this type of perfume, you will need a roll-on cap for your bottle.

For perfume purposes, a light oil such as sweet almond or sunflower works well. Also keep in mind that a carrier oil with a strong scent may influence the perfume. In some cases, it may enhance it. Experiment to find what you like best.

Begin mixing your essential and carrier oils at a 2% dilution by putting 1 teaspoon of carrier oil in a bottle and then adding 2 or 3 drops of your blend. Using another bottle, try a 3% dilution, then decide which you prefer. Because the blend will be used on the body, it is generally considered unsafe to use a dilution ratio higher than 2% or 3%.

Table 7.1 Dilution Amounts

Carrier Oil	1 teaspoon/5 ml	1 tablespoon/15 ml	2 tablespoons/ 30 ml/1 ounce
Essential Oil (2% ratio)	2–3 drops	6–10 drops	12–20 drops
Essential Oil (3% ratio)	3–5 drops	9–16 drops	18–32 drops

As an alternative to a roll-on perfume, you may want to experiment with a solid one. The extra items you will need are beeswax, a small glass bowl, and a decorative container for the finished product.

I find that a 1-ounce bar of beeswax is most economical and easy to measure for recipes because it can be cut into pieces for smaller amounts. Refer to part 7 for more details about beeswax.

Solid Perfume
¼ ounce beeswax

3 tablespoons carrier oil

20–34 drops essential oil blend (2% dilution)

Place the beeswax and carrier oil in a jar in a saucepan of water. Warm it over low heat and gently stir until the wax melts. Remove the jar from the heat and let the mixture cool to room temperature before adding the essential oil. Let it cool completely before using or storing.

If you are wondering about the alcohol in commercial perfumes, it is generally used as an emulsifier to help merge scents. Because it evaporates quickly, it also helps to disperse the scent. Alcohol creates the perfume "trail" that may sometimes linger after a person has left a room. Oil-based perfumes keep the scent on the skin longer and keep it closer to the body, with no trail.

PART THREE

How to Make and Use Medicinal Remedies

In this section, the first chapter provides an overview of healing remedies and methods for applying them. An essential oil diluted in a carrier oil is one of the simplest remedies. Rubbed on sore muscles or added to the bath, they provide soothing relief. Don't overlook the power of the foot bath, where essential oils can help soothe tired feet, fight athlete's foot, and even ease a headache.

If you have ever thought that an ointment, salve, or balm sounds too complicated to make, the straightforward and simple recipes in this section will take you step by step through the process. These recipes are basic guidelines that you may need to adjust for personal preferences or to accommodate any precautions related to the essential oils you use.

Scenting the air not only makes a room smell good but also helps relieve stress, enhance well-being, and much more. Essential oils with antiseptic properties kill airborne bacteria. Because essential oils in the air are absorbed into the body, oils that fight infection or relieve congestion provide a good way to fight colds and flu or treat asthma and bronchitis. To help you get essential oils into the air, a detailed review of the various types of diffusers is included. From simple evaporative diffusers to ultrasonic ones, the information will help you choose the diffuser that is right for you. Details are also included for diffusion methods that you can use on the go.

The second chapter in this section provides an easy-to-use guide for selecting essential oils for a range of ailments and conditions and the methods of treatment that work best. This handy reference will help you get the most from the essential oils you already have and assist you in finding substitutes for ones that you do not currently have on hand.

· · · · · · · ·

CHAPTER 8

❧

Essential Oil Remedies

Like the plants from which they are produced, essential oils are part of the arsenal of home-care remedies. An essential oil diluted in a carrier oil is one of the simplest preparations. Even more so than when mixing scents for perfumes, it is important to keep a record of your remedies. Taking notes will help you determine what adjustments may be needed when repeating a recipe and will help you figure out what works best for you and your family. Whatever type of preparation you make, label it with the date and the ingredients.

As a starting point, table 8.1 provides general guidelines for a 2% dilution ratio of essential oil to carrier oil. While 2% is considered safe for topical applications, use a 1% ratio for children and older adults as well as preparations for use on the face. People with sensitive skin should always use a few less drops of essential oil in their mixtures.

Table 8.1 The 2% Solution

Carrier Oil	Essential Oil
1 teaspoon	2–3 drops
1 tablespoon	6–10 drops
1 fluid ounce	13–20 drops

Essential oils can be used in a range of remedies and methods for treating ailments. The recipes given in this chapter are basic guidelines that you may need to adjust for personal preferences or to accommodate any precautions related to the essential oils you use. Also check the information in part 7 for details about carrier oils and other ingredients, and any precautions for

• • • • • • • •

them. The recipes are given in small amounts, so they are easy to make and allow you to have fresh remedies on hand.

Bath Oils and Salts

In the bath, essential oils help to relieve stress, pain, and muscle aches. A carrier oil provides an even distribution of the essential oil when it is to be used in water. For a healing beauty bath, use milk. The fat in milk acts like a carrier oil to dilute and disperse essential oils. Use 12 to 18 drops of essential oil in an ounce of carrier oil or milk, then add it to your bath.

The milk bath was said to have been a beauty secret of Queen Cleopatra, and modern research has corroborated its effectiveness. Because of milk's high level of lactic acid, dead skin cells are removed, leaving behind a wonderful complexion—all over. Take care whenever you use oils in the bath or shower, as surfaces may become slippery.

In addition to carrier oils and milk, essential oils can be mixed with salts. Coarse sea salt or Epsom salt can be used for a soothing bath. Refer to part 7 for more information on Epsom salt.

Bath Salts

2 cups Epsom or sea salt

2 tablespoons baking soda (optional)

¾ cup carrier oil or blend

1–1½ teaspoons essential oil or blend

Combine the dry ingredients in a glass or ceramic bowl. Mix the carrier and essential oils, then add them to the dry ingredients. Mix thoroughly.

The optional baking soda in the bath salts recipe helps to soothe and soften the skin. This recipe is enough for one or two baths. Add the salts under the running tap just before getting in the tub. If you make a larger amount, store it in a jar with a tight-fitting lid.

Foot Soak

Essential oils diluted in carrier oil or bath salts make a relaxing and therapeutic footbath too. Add 6 to 10 drops of essential oil to a tablespoon of carrier oil and swish into a basin. A warm or hot footbath increases circulation, aids in healing a cold or flu, and helps deal with insomnia. Odd as it may seem, a foot soak helps relieve headaches too. Even soaking your feet in plain warm water helps draw blood down to the feet, which relieves pressure in the head. A cool footbath is a good perk-up on hot summer days when feet can feel sweaty and sore.

Compress

A compress can be hot or cold. Warm compresses relax muscles and soothe aches and pains. They also relieve tension and increase circulation. Cool compresses are used to treat bumps, bruises, sprains, and strains by reducing swelling and inflammation. They also reduce fevers and ease headaches.

Place 6 to 10 drops of essential oil in a tablespoon of carrier oil and add to a quart of hot or cold water. Give the water a good swish before soaking a washcloth in it. Squeeze out the cloth and lay it over the area that needs treatment. Freshen it every ten to fifteen minutes by dipping it in the water again.

Diffusion

Scenting the air is often what comes to mind when we think of aromatherapy. While it is a great way to use essential oils to relieve stress and enhance well-being, there are other benefits. Essential oils with antiseptic properties kill airborne bacteria. Because essential oils in the air are absorbed into the body, oils that fight infection or relieve congestion provide a good way to fight colds and flu or treat asthma and bronchitis. Essential oils can be used to fumigate a sickroom too.

Although a vaporizer works by heating water and creating steam, the terms *vaporizer* and *diffuser* are often used interchangeably. In this book, the word *diffuser* is used for all methods of getting essential oils into the air. Following are details on the various types of diffusers.

Nebulizer

A nebulizer creates a mist or fine spray of tiny droplets. It can put a lot of essential oil into the air quickly. This type of diffuser uses more essential oil than others do. However, most nebulizers have settings and timers that allow you to choose the amount of oil they disperse and set them to run at intervals instead of continuously. Depending on the size of the pump, a nebulizer can be used in large rooms.

Ultrasonic

This type of diffuser creates a fine mist using ultrasonic vibrations. It is basically a humidifier and disperses a smaller amount of essential oil than a nebulizer does. In addition to getting essential oil into the air, the ultrasonic diffuser creates negative ions, which are believed to have health benefits.

Evaporative

Also called a *fan diffuser*, this type of device hastens the process of evaporation by blowing air over a pad or filter onto which essential oils have been applied. While this works well for dispersing scent, it is not the best choice for therapeutic purposes because the lighter components of an essential oil evaporate first, which means you do not get the complete oil all at once.

. . . .

The widely popular *reed diffuser* also disperses scent by evaporation. Although it is effective only in small spaces, when it is placed by a door or window, the scent can be dispersed more quickly. While many reed diffuser kits include chemical-based fragrance oils, making your own with essential oils allows you to choose the scent and decorative container. Details on how to make a reed diffuser are in chapter 11.

Heat

This type of diffuser works by evaporation, using heat to quicken the process. A well-known type called a *candle diffuser* has a small ceramic bowl with space for a tealight candle underneath. You place a few drops of essential oil in the bowl, which is warmed by the candle flame. A drop or two of water can be added to the diffuser bowl to slow the evaporation process. As with the fan diffuser, all of the components of an essential oil are not equally dispersed with a candle diffuser. Some heat diffusers are electric and can be placed on a table or the floor, and others are small plug-ins that sit at the electrical outlet.

On-the-Go Diffusers

Putting essential oil into the air around you isn't limited to the home. No matter how you get around town, you can take a remedy with you.

Inhalers

About the size of a lip balm applicator or a tube of lipstick, a nasal inhaler provides relief on the go. It consists of a tube, a cotton wick, and a screw-on lid. Remove the wick from the tube and place it on a plate. Put about 10 to 15 drops of essential oil or blend onto the wick, then put it back in the tube. For children under the age of ten, use 5 to 8 drops of essential oil. To use an inhaler, place the opened tube under your nose and breathe deeply. Keep the tube tightly closed when not in use. Freshen the wick as needed.

A nasal inhaler is also called a *personal inhaler* or an *aromastick*. It is especially helpful when dealing with a cold or nasal congestion and headaches. A nasal inhaler is also an aid for motion sickness or to combat stress. In addition to being convenient, it also allows you to use essential oils without disturbing people around you.

Plug-Ins

Although some diffusers for the house are small plug-in devices, others are designed for use when not at home. Some plug-ins are small and convenient enough to take on a trip for hotel use, while others are specifically designed for use in the car. There is also a type of plug-in with a USB connector that uses the power of your laptop.

Gel

The base for a homemade gel is aloe. Aloe is a familiar houseplant that is often kept in the kitchen for first aid treatment of burns. Refer to aloe in part 7 for details on what to look for when purchasing the gel and how to harvest it from the plant. Along with the healing power of aloe, essential oils with antiseptic and antibacterial properties work well for making a first aid gel.

Healing Gel

10 drops essential oil or blend

2 tablespoons aloe gel

Add the essential oil to the gel and gently stir until thoroughly mixed. Store in a jar with a tight-fitting lid.

Massage Oil

Creating a massage oil is as easy as adding several drops of essential oil to a carrier oil. Table 8.1 provides guidelines for making a 2% dilution, which is generally appropriate for use on the body. Use a 1% dilution for use on the face for rubbing the temples to ease a headache.

Use firm pressure when massaging muscles and joints, but not so firm that it irritates the skin, exacerbates the pain, or causes discomfort. Gently massaging the stomach can help relieve indigestion. Massaging the stomach and abdomen in a clockwise direction (up on the right, down on the left) can help ease constipation.

Ointments, Salves, and Balms

These three preparations are basically the same but differ in the amount of solidifier used to thicken them. An ointment is the least firm, but it has the advantage of being easy to apply. A salve has a firmer consistency, and a balm is very firm. Unlike a cream, these preparations are not absorbed as quickly and form a protective layer on the skin. In the following recipes, beeswax, shea butter, or cocoa butter can be used as solidifiers. Refer to part 7 for more details on these ingredients. Beeswax forms more of a protective layer than the butters do, but it's worth it to experiment to determine what works best for you. As always, keep careful notes so you can repeat a recipe—or not.

Ointment, Salve, and Balm with Beeswax

½ ounce beeswax

3–8 tablespoons carrier oil or blend

¼–1 teaspoon essential oil or blend (2% dilution)

Place the beeswax and carrier oil in a jar in a saucepan of water. Warm it over low heat, stirring until the wax melts. Remove it from the heat and allow the mixture to cool to room temperature before adding the essential oil. To test the consistency, spoon a little onto a plate and put it in the refrigerator for a minute or two. If you want it firmer, add more beeswax. If it's too thick, add a tiny bit of carrier oil. When you are happy with the consistency of your mixture, let it cool completely, then store in a cool, dark place.

If you like to think in terms of ratios, a 3:1 or 4:1 carrier oil to beeswax ratio tends to work well for a balm. For a salve, try 5:1 or 6:1, and 7:1 or 8:1 for an ointment. Keep in mind that the consistency of your mixture also depends on the viscosity of the oils you use.

Ointment, Salve, and Balm with a Butter

1–3 tablespoons cocoa or shea butter, grated or shaved

1–2 tablespoons carrier oil or blend

12–40 drops essential oil or blend (2% dilution)

Boil a little water in a saucepan and remove it from the heat. Place the butter and carrier oil in a jar in the water. Stir until the butter melts. Remove the jar from the water and allow the mixture to cool to room temperature. Boil the water again, then remove the pan from the heat and place the jar in the water. Stir until any small particles that may have formed have melted. Remove the jar from the water and let the mixture cool again. Add the essential oil and mix thoroughly. Place the jar in the refrigerator for five or six hours. After removing the jar from the fridge, let the mixture come to room temperature before using or storing it.

Again, if you prefer to think in terms of ratios, 1:2 or 1:3 carrier oil to butter works for a balm. Although it usually needs to be scraped up with a fingernail, it begins to melt on contact with the skin. A 1:1 or 1:1½ ratio works for a salve, and 1½:1 or 2:1 works for an ointment. The salve and ointment can be scooped up with a finger. As with beeswax, experiment to find the consistency you like.

Sprays

Whether you want to repel insects or cool menopausal hot flashes, the spray method of topical application works well. It is especially helpful to soothe sunburn or rashes when you don't want to touch your skin. For information about witch hazel and different types of water, refer to part 7.

. . . .

Healing/Cooling Spray

1 teaspoon carrier oil or blend

1 teaspoon essential oil or blend

6 ounces water

1 tablespoon witch hazel

Combine the carrier and essential oils in a spray bottle. Add the water and witch hazel. Shake well before each use.

Steam

Because steam and the antiseptic properties of some essential oils help clear respiratory airways, this is a good way to treat congested sinuses and chest infections. Following are several ways to use steam.

Inhalation Tent

In addition to relieving the congestion of colds, flu, and sinus infections, facial steams are also good for the complexion because they help to deep-clean pores and add moisture to the skin. When adding essential oil to steaming water, use a dropper to avoid getting water vapor in the bottle.

Steam Inhalation

1 quart water

5–8 drops essential oil or blend

Bring the water to a boil. Remove it from the heat and add the essential oils.

Place a bath towel over your head to create a tent above the steaming water. Keep your eyes closed and don't move your face too close to the water. Stay under the tent for about three minutes or until the water cools. If it feels too hot, lift the towel to allow cool air into the tent.

The combination of steam and essential oils can also be used to clean the air of a sickroom or to humidify or freshen a room in winter. Place the steaming saucepan in the room where it is needed. When it cools, reheat it for more steam and add a few more drops of essential oil. To help ease asthma, instead of tenting your head with a towel, use your hand to waft a little of the steam toward your face.

Easy Vapors

A quick way to use steam and essential oils is as easy as making a cup of tea. This also works well if you have asthma.

A Cup of Vapors

1 cup water

1–2 drops essential oil or blend

Boil the water, then pour it into a big mug. Add the essential oil or blend and hold the mug near your face to inhale the vapors.

Shower Steam

Using essential oils in the shower is another quick and easy way to create a steam inhalation. Refer to chapter 11 for details on how to make shower melts. As when using oils in the bath, be careful that the floor of the shower doesn't become slippery.

Simple Steamy Shower

1 washcloth

40–60 drops essential oil or blend

Fold the washcloth in half, sprinkle it with the essential oil, then fold it in half again. Place the washcloth on the floor of the shower under the water stream.

The next chapter contains a quick reference guide to ailments and which essential oils and applications to use to treat them.

CHAPTER 9

❧

Ailments, Oils, and Treatments

This chapter provides a quick reference guide to which essential oils to use for ailments and conditions and which methods of treatment work best. Carrier oils and other ingredients with healing properties are also included. This guide will help you get the most from the essential oils you have on hand. When using the recipes provided in this book, you can refer to this chapter to find substitutes for essential oils that you may not have on hand. Of course, remedies can be made with only one essential oil too.

The remedies covered in chapter 8 can be divided into two basic categories: topical and aromatic.

Topical methods include application using an ointment, salve, or balm; massage; bath, foot soak, or sitz bath; and compress.

Aromatic methods include diffusion in a room with any type of diffuser; direct inhalation a few breaths at a time using a small bottle or an inhaler; and steam as an inhalation to relieve congestion or, as when treating acne, as a cleansing agent.

As previously mentioned, before using any essential oil, it is important to do a patch test on your skin. You may also want to discuss using essential oils with your doctor, especially if you are on any type of medication, have a medical condition, or are pregnant.

Table 9.1 Ailments, Methods of Treatment, Essential Oils, and Other Ingredients

---

Acne

Methods: Steam, topical application

Essential Oils: Bergamot, cajeput, cedarwood, chamomile, clary sage, geranium, grapefruit, helichrysum, juniper berry, lavender, lemon, lemongrass, lime, mandarin, manuka, niaouli, palmarosa, patchouli, peppermint, petitgrain, rosemary, sage, sandalwood, spearmint, tea tree, thyme, vetiver, ylang-ylang

Carrier Oils: Rosehip seed, sunflower

Other Ingredient: Aloe vera

Anxiety

Methods: Bath, diffusion, inhaler, massage

Essential Oils: Amyris, angelica, anise seed, basil, bergamot, black pepper, cardamom, cedarwood (Virginia), chamomile, citronella, clary sage, clove bud, coriander, frankincense, geranium, hyssop, juniper berry, lavender, lemon balm, manuka, marjoram, neroli, orange, palmarosa, patchouli, petitgrain, rose, spearmint, vetiver, ylang-ylang

---

Arthritis

Methods: Bath, compress, massage

Essential Oils: Angelica, anise seed, basil, bay laurel, black pepper, cajeput, carrot seed, cedarwood, chamomile, cinnamon leaf, clove bud, coriander, cypress, eucalyptus (blue), fennel, fir needle, ginger, helichrysum, hyssop, juniper berry, lavender, lemon, lime, marjoram, myrrh, niaouli, pine, ravintsara, rosemary, sage, thyme, vetiver

Other Ingredient: Epsom salt

Asthma

Methods: Diffusion, steam

Essential Oils: Cajeput, caraway seed, clary sage, clove bud, cypress, eucalyptus, fennel, frankincense, helichrysum, hyssop, lavender, lemon, lemon balm, lime, marjoram, myrrh, niaouli, peppermint, pine, ravintsara, rose, rosemary, sage, spearmint, tea tree, thyme

Note: When dealing with asthma, always use smaller amounts in diffusers. Also refer to the special instructions for steam inhalation in chapter 8.

Athlete's Foot

Methods: Footbath, topical application

Essential Oils: Bay laurel, cajeput, cedarwood (Atlas), clove bud, eucalyptus (lemon), lavender, lemongrass, manuka, myrrh, palmarosa, patchouli, tea tree

Table 9.1 Ailments, Methods of Treatment, Essential Oils, and Other Ingredients (*continued*)

Blisters   *Method:* Topical application   *Essential Oils:* Bergamot, eucalyptus (blue), lavender, lemon, myrrh, tea tree
Boils   *Methods:* Bath, compress, topical application   *Essential Oils:* Bergamot, caraway seed, chamomile, clary sage, eucalyptus (blue), frankincense, helichrysum, lavender, lemon, lime, myrrh, niaouli, patchouli, sage, sandalwood, tea tree
Bronchitis   *Methods:* Diffusion, inhaler, steam, topical application (chest rub)   *Essential Oils:* Angelica, anise seed, basil, cajeput, caraway seed, cedarwood, cinnamon leaf, clove bud, cypress, elemi, eucalyptus (blue), fennel, fir needle, frankincense, helichrysum, hyssop, lavender, lemon, lemon balm, lime, marjoram, myrrh, niaouli, orange, peppermint, pine, ravintsara, rosemary, sandalwood, spearmint, tea tree, thyme
Bruises   *Methods:* Compress, topical application   *Essential Oils:* Bay laurel, clove bud, fennel, geranium, helichrysum, hyssop, lavender, marjoram, palmarosa, rose, thyme   *Other Ingredients:* Epsom salt, witch hazel
Burns   *Methods:* Bath, compress, topical application   *Essential Oils:* Carrot seed, chamomile, clove bud, eucalyptus (blue), geranium, helichrysum, lavender, niaouli, tea tree, thyme   *Carrier Oils:* Calendula, St. John's wort   *Other Ingredients:* Aloe vera, cocoa butter
Bursitis   *Methods:* Compress, massage   *Essential Oils:* Cajeput, cypress, eucalyptus (blue), ginger, helichrysum, juniper berry, marjoram
Cellulite   *Methods:* Bath, massage   *Essential Oils:* Cypress, fennel, geranium, grapefruit, juniper berry, lemon, lime, thyme

. . . .

Table 9.1 Ailments, Methods of Treatment, Essential Oils, and Other Ingredients (*continued*)

Chapped Skin
Methods: Bath, topical application
Essential Oils: Helichrysum, lavender, myrrh, neroli, palmarosa, patchouli, rose
Carrier Oils: Coconut, evening primrose, sesame
Other Ingredients: Aloe vera, beeswax, cocoa butter, shea butter
Chicken Pox
Methods: Bath, compress, topical application
Essential Oils: Bergamot, chamomile (German), clove bud, eucalyptus, manuka, ravintsara, tea tree
Chilblains
Methods: Steam, topical application
Essential Oils: Black pepper, chamomile, lavender, lemon, lime, marjoram
Circulation
Method: Massage
Essential Oils: Basil, black pepper, cajeput, cinnamon leaf, coriander, cypress, eucalyptus (blue), geranium, ginger, grapefruit, lemon, lemongrass, lime, niaouli, pine, rose, rosemary, sage, thyme, vetiver
Cold Sores
Methods: Steam, topical application
Essential Oils: Bergamot, eucalyptus, hyssop, lemon, lime, manuka, ravintsara, tea tree
Colds
Methods: Bath, diffusion, inhaler, steam
Essential Oils: Angelica, anise seed, basil, bay laurel, bergamot, black pepper, cajeput, caraway seed, cedarwood, cinnamon leaf, citronella, clove bud, coriander, cypress, elemi, eucalyptus, fir needle, frankincense, ginger, grapefruit, helichrysum, hyssop, juniper berry, lavender, lemon, lemongrass, lime, manuka, marjoram, myrrh, neroli, niaouli, orange, peppermint, pine, ravintsara, rosemary, sage, spearmint, tea tree, thyme
Constipation
Methods: Bath, compress, massage
Essential Oils: Black pepper, cardamom, fennel, ginger, mandarin, marjoram, neroli, orange, peppermint, pine
Corns and Calluses
Method: Topical application
Essential Oils: Carrot seed, lemon, lime, myrrh

Table 9.1 Ailments, Methods of Treatment, Essential Oils, and Other Ingredients (*continued*)

Coughs

Methods: Diffusion, inhaler, steam

Essential Oils: Angelica, anise seed, basil, cajeput, caraway seed, cedarwood, cinnamon leaf, clary sage, clove bud, coriander, cypress, elemi, eucalyptus (blue), fennel, fir needle, frankincense, ginger, helichrysum, hyssop, lavender, lemon, lemon balm, lime, manuka, marjoram, myrrh, niaouli, orange, peppermint, pine, ravintsara, rosemary, sage, sandalwood, spearmint, tea tree, thyme

---

Cuts and Scrapes

Methods: Compress, topical application

Essential Oils: Bergamot, caraway seed, carrot seed, chamomile, clove bud, cypress, elemi, eucalyptus, frankincense, geranium, helichrysum, hyssop, lavender, lemon, lime, manuka, myrrh, niaouli, patchouli, pine, rosemary, sage, sandalwood, tea tree, thyme, vetiver

Carrier Oils: Calendula, sesame, St. John's wort

Other Ingredients: Aloe vera, witch hazel

Depression

Methods: Diffusion, inhaler, massage

Essential Oils: Basil, bergamot, chamomile (Roman), cinnamon leaf, citronella, clary sage, geranium, ginger, grapefruit, helichrysum, lavender, lemon balm, neroli, patchouli, peppermint, petitgrain, rose, vetiver, ylang-ylang

---

Dermatitis

Methods: Bath, compress, topical application

Essential Oils: Carrot seed, cedarwood (Atlas), chamomile, geranium, helichrysum, hyssop, juniper berry, lavender, palmarosa, patchouli, peppermint, rose, rosemary, sage, spearmint, thyme

Carrier Oils: Avocado, borage, coconut

Other Ingredient: Cocoa butter

Earaches

Method: Compress

Essential Oils: Basil, cajeput, chamomile, lavender, thyme

Table 9.1 Ailments, Methods of Treatment, Essential Oils, and Other Ingredients (*continued*)

Eczema

Methods: Bath, topical application

Essential Oils: Bay laurel, bergamot, cajeput, carrot seed, cedarwood, chamomile, geranium, helichrysum, hyssop, juniper berry, lavender, lemon balm, myrrh, palmarosa, patchouli, rose, rosemary, sage, thyme

Carrier Oils: Almond, avocado, borage, coconut, evening primrose, rosehip seed, St. John's wort, sunflower

Other Ingredients: Cocoa butter, shea butter, witch hazel

Edema

Methods: Bath, massage

Essential Oils: Carrot seed, cypress, fennel, geranium

Fainting

Method: Inhaler

Essential Oils: Basil, black pepper, neroli, peppermint, rosemary

---

Fever

Methods: Bath, compress

Essential Oils: Basil, bay laurel, bergamot, black pepper, chamomile (Roman), cinnamon leaf, citronella, eucalyptus, fir needle, ginger, helichrysum, lemon, lemon balm, lemongrass, lime, niaouli, orange, palmarosa, patchouli, peppermint, sage, spearmint, tea tree

---

Flu

Methods: Bath, diffusion, inhaler, steam

Essential Oils: Anise seed, basil, bay laurel, bergamot, black pepper, cajeput, cinnamon leaf, citronella, clove bud, coriander, cypress, eucalyptus (blue), fir needle, frankincense, ginger, grapefruit, helichrysum, hyssop, juniper berry, lavender, lemon, lemongrass, lime, manuka, neroli, niaouli, orange, peppermint, pine, ravintsara, rosemary, sage, spearmint, tea tree, thyme

---

Gout

Methods: Bath, massage

Essential Oils: Angelica, basil, carrot seed, coriander, juniper berry, lemon, pine, rosemary, thyme

---

Hangover

Methods: Diffusion, inhaler

Essential Oils: Anise seed, cardamom, ginger, grapefruit, juniper berry, lemon, mandarin, peppermint, pine, spearmint, thyme

---

• • • • • • • •

Table 9.1 Ailments, Methods of Treatment, Essential Oils, and Other Ingredients (*continued*)

Hay Fever *Methods:* Bath, massage, diffusion, inhaler, steam *Essential Oils:* Chamomile, citronella, clove bud, eucalyptus (blue), lemon balm, manuka, ravintsara, rose
Head Lice *Method:* Topical application *Essential Oils:* Cajeput, cinnamon leaf, citronella, eucalyptus (blue), geranium, lavender, lemongrass, pine, rosemary, tea tree, thyme
Headaches *Methods:* Compress, diffusion, inhaler, massage *Essential Oils:* Angelica, basil, cajeput, cardamom, chamomile, citronella, clary sage, coriander, elemi, eucalyptus (blue), grapefruit, lavender, lemon, lemon balm, lemongrass, manuka, marjoram, neroli, niaouli, orange, patchouli, peppermint, petitgrain, rose, rosemary, sage, spearmint, thyme
Hemorrhoids Methods: Bath, topical application *Essential Oils:* Cypress, frankincense, geranium, juniper berry, myrrh *Other Ingredients:* Aloe vera, beeswax, witch hazel
Indigestion *Method:* Massage *Essential Oils:* Angelica, anise seed, bay laurel, black pepper, caraway seed, cardamom, carrot seed, chamomile, coriander, fennel, ginger, hyssop, lavender, lemon balm, lemongrass, mandarin, marjoram, myrrh, orange, peppermint, petitgrain, rosemary, sage, spearmint
Inflammation *Method:* Topical application *Essential Oils:* Chamomile, citronella, elemi, fennel, frankincense, helichrysum, hyssop, lavender, lemon balm, neroli, orange, peppermint, rose, sage, tea tree, thyme, vetiver *Carrier Oils:* Apricot, borage, coconut, hazel, jojoba, rosehip seed, sesame, St. John's wort, sunflower *Other Ingredient:* Epsom salt

Table 9.1 Ailments, Methods of Treatment, Essential Oils, and Other Ingredients (*continued*)

Insect Bites and Stings

Method: Topical application

Essential Oils: Basil, bergamot, cajeput, chamomile, cinnamon leaf, citronella, eucalyptus, lavender, lemon, lemon balm, lemongrass, lime, manuka, niaouli, patchouli, peppermint, spearmint, tea tree, thyme, ylang-ylang

Other Ingredients: Shea butter, witch hazel

Insomnia

Methods: Bath, diffusion, massage

Essential Oils: Basil, chamomile, clary sage, lavender, lemon balm, mandarin, marjoram, neroli, orange, petitgrain, ravintsara, rose, sandalwood, spearmint, thyme, vetiver, ylang-ylang

---

Jet Lag

Method: Diffusion

Essential Oils: Bergamot, geranium, ginger, lemon, lemongrass, neroli, peppermint, rosemary

---

Jock Itch

Methods: Bath, topical application

Essential Oils: Bay laurel, lemongrass, manuka, tea tree

Laryngitis

Methods: Diffusion, steam

Essential Oils: Bergamot, cajeput, caraway seed, clary sage, eucalyptus (lemon), frankincense, lavender, myrrh, pine, ravintsara, sage, thyme

---

Lumbago

Methods: Bath, massage

Essential Oils: Clove bud, eucalyptus (blue), marjoram

Menopausal Discomfort

Methods: Bath, diffusion, massage, spray

Essential Oils: Anise seed, chamomile, clary sage, coriander, cypress, fennel, geranium, lavender, neroli, palmarosa, patchouli, rose, sage, spearmint, thyme, vetiver, ylang-ylang

---

Menstrual Cramps

Methods: Bath, compress, massage

Essential Oils: Anise seed, chamomile, cinnamon leaf, clary sage, coriander, ginger, lavender, lemon balm, marjoram, patchouli, rose, rosemary, sage, thyme

---

Table 9.1 Ailments, Methods of Treatment, Essential Oils, and Other Ingredients (*continued*)

Migraines

Methods: Compress, diffusion, inhaler

Essential Oils: Angelica, basil, chamomile (Roman), citronella, clary sage, coriander, lavender, lemon balm, manuka, marjoram, peppermint, spearmint

Motion Sickness

Method: Inhaler

Essential Oils: Chamomile, ginger, peppermint, spearmint

Muscle Aches and Pains

Methods: Bath, compress, massage

Essential Oils: Amyris, anise seed, basil, black pepper, cajeput, chamomile, cinnamon leaf, clary sage, clove bud, coriander, cypress, eucalyptus (blue), fir needle, ginger, helichrysum, juniper berry, lavender, lemongrass, manuka, marjoram, niaouli, peppermint, pine, ravintsara, rosemary, sage, spearmint, thyme, vetiver

Carrier Oil: St. John's wort

Other Ingredient: Epsom salt

Nail Fungus

Method: Topical application

Essential Oils: Clove bud, eucalyptus (lemon), ravintsara, tea tree

Nausea

Methods: Diffusion, inhaler

Essential Oils: Anise seed, basil, black pepper, cardamom, chamomile, clove bud, coriander, fennel, ginger, grapefruit, lavender, lemon balm, mandarin, marjoram, orange, peppermint, rose, spearmint

Poison Ivy

Method: Topical application

Essential Oils: Chamomile, cypress, frankincense, helichrysum, lavender, myrrh, peppermint, tea tree

Premenstrual Syndrome (PMS)

Methods: Bath, diffusion, massage

Essential Oils: Bergamot, caraway seed, cardamom, carrot seed, chamomile, clary sage, coriander, cypress, fennel, frankincense, geranium, grapefruit, lavender, lemon balm, marjoram, neroli, palmarosa, rose, vetiver, ylang-ylang

· · · · · · · ·

Table 9.1 Ailments, Methods of Treatment, Essential Oils, and Other Ingredients (*continued*)

Psoriasis
Methods: Bath, topical application
Essential Oils: Angelica, bay laurel, bergamot, carrot seed, cedarwood (Virginia), chamomile, juniper berry, lavender, rose
Carrier Oils: Borage, coconut, evening primrose, rosehip seed, St. John's wort
Other Ingredients: Cocoa butter, Epsom salt, shea butter, witch hazel
Rashes
Methods: Bath, compress, topical application
Essential Oils: Bay laurel, bergamot, carrot seed, cedarwood (Virginia), chamomile, clary sage, elemi, helichrysum, lavender, myrrh, palmarosa, peppermint, sandalwood, tea tree
Carrier Oils: Almond, apricot, borage, hazel, jojoba, olive, sesame
Ringworm
Method: Topical application
Essential Oils: Geranium, lavender, manuka, myrrh, peppermint
Scabies
Method: Bath
Essential Oils: Bergamot, cajeput, cinnamon leaf, lavender, lemongrass, peppermint, pine, rosemary, thyme
Other Ingredient: Aloe vera
Scars
Method: Topical application
Essential Oils: Elemi, frankincense, helichrysum, lavender, mandarin, neroli, niaouli, palmarosa, patchouli, rose
Carrier Oils: Borage, calendula, coconut, olive, rosehip seed, sunflower
Other Ingredient: Cocoa butter
Sciatica
Methods: Bath, massage
Essential Oils: Marjoram, pine, thyme
Seasonal Affective Disorder (SAD)
Methods: Bath, diffusion
Essential Oils: Bergamot, ginger, grapefruit, lemon balm, orange, petitgrain, ylang-ylang
Shingles
Methods: Bath, topical application
Essential Oils: Clove bud, geranium, ravintsara, tea tree

• • • • • • • •

Table 9.1 Ailments, Methods of Treatment, Essential Oils, and Other Ingredients (*continued*)

Sinus Infection   *Method:* Steam   *Essential Oils:* Basil, cajeput, cedarwood (Virginia), elemi, eucalyptus, fir needle, ginger, manuka, niaouli, peppermint, pine, ravintsara, sandalwood, spearmint, tea tree, thyme
Sore Throat   *Methods:* Diffusion, steam   *Essential Oils:* Bay laurel, bergamot, cajeput, caraway seed, chamomile (Roman), clary sage, eucalyptus, geranium, ginger, hyssop, lavender, myrrh, niaouli, pine, spearmint, thyme
Sprains and Strains   *Methods:* Compress, massage   *Essential Oils:* Bay laurel, black pepper, chamomile, clove bud, eucalyptus (blue), ginger, helichrysum, lavender, lemongrass, marjoram, pine, rosemary, thyme, vetiver   *Other Ingredients:* Epsom salt, witch hazel
Stress   *Methods:* Bath, diffusion, inhaler, massage   *Essential Oils:* Amyris, angelica, anise seed, basil, bergamot, black pepper, cardamom, cedarwood, chamomile, cinnamon leaf, citronella, clary sage, clove bud, coriander, cypress, elemi, fir needle, frankincense, geranium, grapefruit, helichrysum, hyssop, juniper berry, lavender, lemon balm, lemongrass, mandarin, manuka, marjoram, neroli, orange, palmarosa, patchouli, peppermint, petitgrain, pine, ravintsara, rose, rosemary, sage, sandalwood, spearmint, thyme, vetiver, ylang-ylang
Stretch Marks   *Method:* Topical application   *Essential Oils:* Elemi, frankincense, helichrysum, lavender, mandarin, myrrh, neroli, palmarosa, patchouli, rose   *Carrier Oils:* Borage, coconut, olive, rosehip seed   *Other Ingredients:* Beeswax, cocoa butter, shea butter
Sunburn   *Method:* Topical application   *Essential Oils:* Carrot seed, chamomile, geranium, helichrysum, lavender, lemon balm, peppermint, spearmint   *Carrier Oils:* Avocado, calendula, coconut, St. John's wort, sunflower   *Other Ingredients:* Aloe vera, cocoa butter

Table 9.1 Ailments, Methods of Treatment, Essential Oils, and Other Ingredients (*continued*)

Tendonitis
Methods: Compress, massage
Essential Oils: Black pepper, cypress, lemongrass, pine, rosemary, vetiver
Tonsillitis
Method: Steam
Essential Oils: Bay laurel, bergamot, chamomile (Roman), geranium, hyssop, thyme
Vaginal Infection
Method: Sitz bath
Essential Oils: Cajeput, lemongrass, manuka, myrrh, palmarosa, tea tree
Varicose Veins
Methods: Compress, massage
Essential Oils: Bergamot, cypress, fennel, grapefruit, lemon, lemongrass, lime, rosemary, sage
Other Ingredient: Witch hazel
Vertigo
Method: Inhaler
Essential Oils: Anise seed, ginger, lavender, neroli, peppermint
Warts
Method: Topical application
Essential Oils: Cajeput, cedarwood (Virginia), cinnamon leaf, lemon, lime, manuka, tea tree
Whooping Cough
Method: Steam
Essential Oils: Anise seed, clary sage, cypress, helichrysum, hyssop, lavender, manuka, niaouli, ravintsara, rosemary, tea tree

In the next section, we will explore how to use essential oils for personal care, emotional support, and spiritual enhancement.

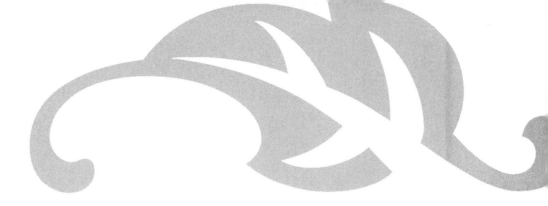

PART FOUR

Personal Care and Well-Being

Moving beyond remedies for treating ailments, this section provides information on making your own skin and hair care products. By making your own, you can reduce or eliminate the amount of chemicals you use on your body. With essential oils, you can create special scents for products that are uniquely your own. If you're in a hurry, add them to organic unscented creams or lotions.

We will see how some health care remedies and methods also work for beauty care. In addition to essential oils, this section covers some of the dos and don'ts especially when it comes to facial scrubs and masks. Preparations to help keep hair clean and healthy are also included, as well as some body care products. A table listing the appropriate essential and carrier oils and other ingredients is included for each type of personal care product to help you choose the ones that will work best for you.

Another chapter covers the classic aromatherapy use of scent. Because the sense of smell is intimately linked with memory and emotion, essential oils provide a powerful treatment and enhancement for the emotions. They can help reduce stress, calm anxiety, alter moods, focus attention, and more.

This section also explores the chakra system and how these energy centers are associated with various aspects of life. We will see how essential oils can be used to activate and move chakra energy to foster and maintain balance. Because scent has been an integral part of religious practices since ancient times, details are included for making scented candles to enhance and support spirituality. With fire regarded as the element of transformation, we will see how to use a little candle magic to initiate change in our lives.

CHAPTER 10

❧

Personal Care Products

Just as essential oils provide us with natural healing through home remedies, they also provide the means to eliminate or at least reduce the amount of chemicals we use on our bodies. In addition, by using essential oils, we can create special scents for products that are uniquely our own. Essential oils can also be added to organic unscented creams or lotions.

Skin Care

Good skin starts by being clean. Always remove makeup and wash your face at the end of the day. Also wash your face before using a facial scrub or mask or before applying moisturizer. Both a scrub and a mask exfoliate and smooth the skin. While a mask provides deeper cleansing, it needs to be used carefully by those with dry or sensitive skin.

The steam inhalation mentioned in chapter 8 for treating colds, bronchitis, and other ailments is also good for the skin. It not only opens and cleanses the pores but also hydrates the skin. A facial steam is good for most skin types but should be avoided if your complexion is prone to thread veins, which are fine red lines on the cheeks.

Face Scrubs

Cornmeal or oatmeal is commonly used for the base of a facial scrub. Both will exfoliate; however, oatmeal is a little gentler and can be used on sensitive skin. Oatmeal also aids in moisturizing the skin. Even though cornmeal helps to get rid of excess oil, it won't dry out the skin. When using cornmeal, look for organic, non-GMO products. For oatmeal, look for organic. (The oat market is not large enough to interest GMO production.)

Exfoliating Facial Scrub

2–3 drops carrier oil

1–2 drops essential oil

1 teaspoon finely ground cornmeal or oatmeal

Combine the carrier and essential oils, then add them to the meal and mix well. Add another drop or two of carrier oil if necessary to hold the mixture together. Gently massage it over your face. Rinse with lukewarm water.

As an alternative to the carrier oil in the recipe, a little honey or yogurt can be used to moisten the mixture. Although a face scrub is good for the complexion, it should not be used more than once a week, as too much exfoliation may damage the skin.

Face Mask

A face mask cleanses, nourishes, and stimulates the skin. One of the base ingredients for a mask is flour; oat or rice is best. If you have oatmeal, use a food processor to grind it into a fine powder. Oat is good for all skin types, even sensitive, and with anti-inflammatory properties it helps to soothe any irritation. It also helps to remove dirt from pores and moisturize the skin. Rice flour also has anti-inflammatory properties and absorbs oils. Look for organic oat flour or oatmeal. When using rice flour, look for organic, non-GMO.

The other popular base for a mask is cosmetic clay. Because of its high mineral content, clay rejuvenates the skin. Three widely used clays are bentonite, French green clay, and white kaolin. Bentonite clay is highly absorbent, healing, and suitable for oily skin. French green clay is also highly absorbent. It shrinks pore size and is suitable for oily skin. White kaolin is absorbent but mild and is suitable for normal, dry, and sensitive skin types. It is also called white cosmetic clay and china clay.

Although a great deal has been written about whether a mask should dry on the face, recent consensus among beauty experts is not to let it dry. If you have had a mask dry on your face, you may remember your skin feeling tight. This is not because it shrank the pores; it's because the mask sucked the moisture out of your skin. The best time to remove a facial mask is just when it begins to dry.

Cleansing Face Mask

2 tablespoons oat or rice flour or clay

1 tablespoon honey, yogurt, or milk (or just enough to make a paste)

6–10 drops essential oil or blend

· · · · · · · ·

Combine all ingredients and mix well. Apply to the face close to hairline, lips, and eyes. Be careful not to touch the eyes. When it begins to dry, rinse thoroughly with warm water, pat dry, and apply a moisturizer.

Moisturizers

The daily use of a moisturizer is important, and even more so immediately following a facial scrub or mask.

Simple Oil Moisturizer

4 tablespoons carrier oil or blend

12–20 drops essential oil or blend for a facial moisturizer

or 24–40 drops essential oil or blend for a body moisturizer

Combine the oils, mix thoroughly, and apply with fingertips. Store in a bottle with a tight-fitting lid.

Butter-Based Moisturizer

2 tablespoons cocoa or shea butter, grated or shaved

1½ tablespoons carrier oil or blend

15–20 drops essential oil or blend for a facial moisturizer

or 18–30 drops essential oil or blend for a body moisturizer

Boil a little water in a saucepan and remove it from the heat. Place the butter and carrier oil in a jar in the saucepan of water. Stir until the butter melts. Remove the jar from the water, let the mixture cool to room temperature, and then reheat. After the mixture cools again, add the essential oil and mix thoroughly. Place the jar in the refrigerator for five or six hours. Remove it from the fridge and let it come to room temperature before using or storing.

Whether or not small particles precipitate from the butter after the first warming, heating it a second time gives the mixture a smooth texture.

Toners and Astringents

Both toners and astringents are used after washing the face and before moisturizing. A toner hydrates as it further cleans the skin, removing any residue. An astringent also cleans and helps to remove excess oil. Toners are generally good for all types of skin. While best for oily skin, an astringent can be used on other complexions to remove excess dirt and shrink pores; however, it should not be used every day. Although flower water, such as rose or lavender, is often used as the base of a toner or astringent, chamomile or other herb tea works well too. Let the tea cool before making the preparation. During the summer, keep the toner or astringent in the fridge for a refreshing pick-me-up.

Facial Astringent
¼ cup flower water or herb tea
15–25 drops essential oil or blend
1 tablespoon witch hazel

Facial Toner
¼ cup flower water or herb tea
12–20 drops essential oil or blend

When using tea, let it steep for fifteen minutes and then cool. Combine all ingredients in a bottle and shake well. Apply to the face with a cotton ball.

Table 10.1 Essential Oils and Other Ingredients for Skin Care

Combination Skin

Essential Oils: Cajeput, chamomile, elemi, lavender, lemon balm, marjoram, neroli, palmarosa, patchouli, petitgrain, rose, spearmint, vetiver, ylang-ylang

Carrier Oils: Almond, apricot, borage, coconut, hazel, jojoba, rosehip seed, sunflower

Dry Skin

Essential Oils: Chamomile, elemi, frankincense, geranium, lavender, lemon balm, myrrh, neroli, palmarosa, patchouli, rose, vetiver, ylang-ylang

Carrier Oils: Almond, apricot, avocado, borage, calendula, coconut, evening primrose, hazel, jojoba, olive, rosehip seed, sesame, sunflower

Other Ingredients: Beeswax, cocoa butter, shea butter

Mature Skin

Essential Oils: Amyris, carrot seed, chamomile, clary sage, elemi, fennel, frankincense, geranium, helichrysum, lavender, lemon balm, mandarin, myrrh, neroli, palmarosa, patchouli, rose, vetiver, ylang-ylang

Carrier Oils: Almond, apricot, avocado, borage, calendula, coconut, evening primrose, hazel, jojoba, olive, rosehip seed, sesame, sunflower

Other Ingredients: Beeswax, cocoa butter, shea butter

Normal Skin

Essential Oils: Amyris, angelica, chamomile, elemi, lavender, lemon balm, lemongrass, marjoram, neroli, palmarosa, patchouli, peppermint, petitgrain, rose, spearmint, vetiver, ylang-ylang

Carrier Oils: Almond, apricot, borage, coconut, hazel, jojoba, rosehip seed, sunflower

Other Ingredients: Beeswax, cocoa butter

· · · · · · · ·

Table 10.1 Essential Oils and Other Ingredients for Skin Care (*continued*)

Oily Skin

Essential Oils: Bergamot, cajeput, caraway seed, cedarwood, chamomile, citronella, clary sage, coriander, cypress, eucalyptus, elemi, fennel, geranium, grapefruit, helichrysum, juniper berry, lavender, lemon, lemon balm, lemongrass, lime, mandarin, manuka, neroli, niaouli, orange, palmarosa, patchouli, peppermint, petitgrain, rose, rosemary, sandalwood, spearmint, tea tree, thyme, vetiver, ylang-ylang

Carrier Oils: Almond, apricot, borage, coconut, hazel, jojoba, rosehip seed, sunflower

Other Ingredients: Aloe vera, beeswax, shea butter, witch hazel

Pimple Outbreaks

Essential Oils: Amyris, bergamot, cajeput, cedarwood, clary sage, helichrysum, lavender, lemon, lemon balm, lime, mandarin, manuka, niaouli, orange, palmarosa, petitgrain, sandalwood, spearmint, tea tree, thyme

Carrier Oils: Borage, hazel, rosehip seed

Other Ingredients: Beeswax, shea butter, witch hazel

Sensitive Skin

Essential Oils: Angelica, chamomile, lavender, neroli, rose, spearmint

Carrier Oils: Almond, apricot

Other Ingredients: Beeswax, cocoa butter

Wrinkles and Fine Lines

Essential Oils: Amyris, carrot seed, clary sage, elemi, frankincense, geranium, mandarin, myrrh, neroli, palmarosa, patchouli, rose

Carrier Oils: Borage, jojoba, rosehip seed, sunflower

Other Ingredient: Beeswax

Hair Care

Hair usually takes a beating from frequent shampooing, lots of sun in the summer, and tinkering with the color. While we often realize that we abuse our hair and try to compensate, we almost totally forget about the scalp. Healthy hair starts with a healthy scalp, and to repair the damage we may have done to our hair, we need to take care of both.

A scalp massage improves blood circulation, which promotes healthy hair growth. It also helps to remove dandruff and prevent it from reforming.

Scalp Massage Oil

1 tablespoon carrier oil or blend

3–5 drops essential oil or blend

Combine the oils. Before shampooing, put a few drops on your fingertips and massage into your scalp. Store any leftover oil in a bottle with a tight-fitting cap.

While coconut oil is revered for conditioning and reviving hair, other carrier oils work well too. For more details on cocoa and shea butters, refer to part 7.

Hair Conditioner

1 teaspoon cocoa or shea butter

3 tablespoons carrier oil or blend

12–20 drops essential oil or blend

Boil a little water in a saucepan and remove it from the heat. Place the butter and carrier oil in a jar in the water. Stir until everything melts together. Allow the mixture to cool to room temperature, then repeat the heating process. Let it cool to room temperature again and add the essential oils. Place the jar in the refrigerator for several hours until the mixture sets, then let it come to room temperature. Use a fingerful of the conditioner to massage into the scalp and work through the hair. Wrap with a towel for fifteen to thirty minutes. Shampoo and rinse well.

Dandruff

Dandruff can have several causes, including dry or oily skin, a skin condition, or even stress. Essential oils come to the rescue, and if stress is part of the cause, include calming scents in your dandruff blend. Keeping the scalp and hair clean and getting some sun on a regular basis helps to keep dandruff in check.

Soothing Dandruff Blend

2 tablespoons carrier oil or blend

8–10 drops essential oil or blend

Combine the oils, then massage gently into the scalp. Leave the mixture on for about fifteen minutes. Shampoo and rinse well.

Table 10.2 Essential Oils and Other Ingredients for Hair Care

Dandruff

Essential Oils: Bay laurel, cardamom, cedarwood (Atlas), clary sage, eucalyptus, geranium, lavender, lemon, lime, mandarin, manuka, marjoram, myrrh, patchouli, peppermint, rosemary, sage, spearmint, tea tree, ylang-ylang

Carrier Oils: Avocado, coconut, jojoba, olive, sesame

Other Ingredient: Aloe vera

Dry Hair

Essential Oils: Bay laurel, clary sage, geranium, myrrh

Carrier Oils: Almond, apricot, avocado, coconut, hazelnut, jojoba, olive

Other Ingredients: Cocoa butter, shea butter

Normal Hair

Essential Oils: Carrot seed, geranium, lavender, lemon, rosemary

Carrier Oils: Coconut, jojoba

Oily Hair

Essential Oils: Bay laurel, caraway seed, cedarwood, citronella, clary sage, cypress, grapefruit, juniper berry, lemon, lime, manuka, niaouli, patchouli, petitgrain, tea tree, ylang-ylang

Carrier Oils: Almond, apricot, hazelnut, jojoba

Hair Growth

Essential Oils: Basil, cedarwood (Atlas), cypress, grapefruit, lavender, neroli, rosemary, sage, thyme, ylang-ylang

Carrier Oils: Almond, avocado

Body Care

In addition to being costly, most commercial body care products contain chemicals. Not only that, but when using various products, we can end up with competing fragrances. By making our own preparations, we can get away from chemicals and create an ensemble of preparations with our favorite scents.

Body Scrub and Bath Bombs

Unlike a scrub for the face, a body scrub does not need to be as gentle unless you have a skin condition that could be exacerbated. The base of a body scrub is sugar and Epsom or sea salt. Salts contain minerals that are good for the skin. Sugar is used to soften the abrasiveness of the salt. If you have sensitive skin, use sugar without salt.

· · · · · · · ·

Body Scrub

½ cup granulated sugar (white or brown)

½ cup Epsom or sea salt

5 tablespoons carrier oil or blend

1 teaspoon essential oil or blend

Combine the dry ingredients in a bowl. Mix the carrier and essential oils, then blend all the ingredients together. Store in a jar with a tight-fitting lid.

In addition to adding essential oils to bathwater or bath salts, as mentioned in chapter 8, bath bombs can add a little fun to regular body care. The ingredient citric acid provides the fizz. Refer to part 7 for details on what to consider when buying citric acid.

Bath Bombs

1 cup baking soda

½ cup citric acid

1 teaspoon dried herbs and/or flower petals (optional)

½ teaspoon cocoa or shea butter

10 drops essential oil or blend

1–2 drops carrier oil (if necessary)

Mix the dry ingredients and set aside. Boil a little water in a saucepan, then remove it from the heat. Place the cocoa or shea butter in a jar in the water and stir until melted. Let it cool, then stir in the essential oils. Slowly add the dry ingredients until the consistency of the mixture is like clumpy wet sand. If the mixture is too dry and crumbly, add a drop or two of carrier oil to hold it together. Press the mixture into decorative candy molds and let them sit for a day or two before storing.

As an alternative to candy molds, use a melon baller to shape the bath bombs. Let the balls sit on a piece of wax paper for a day or two before using or storing.

Body Powder

After creating a luxurious blend of scents for the bath, follow it with a matching or complementary body powder. The base for a powder can be cornstarch, arrowroot, or finely ground rice or oat flour. When using cornstarch or rice flour, look for organic, non-GMO products. Also look for organic oat flour or unsulfured arrowroot. You may want to experiment with different combinations of base powders to find a texture you like.

• • • • • • • •

Simple Body Powder

1 cup base powder

¼ cup baking soda or white kaolin clay

½–¾ teaspoon essential oil or blend

Combine the dry ingredients and add the essential oil. Mix thoroughly with a fork or small egg whisk to break up any clumps. Store in a decorative jar with a tight-fitting lid.

Deodorant

Since bacteria is the cause of body odor, what better way to deal with it than with bacteria-fighting essential oils such as cardamom, cypress, juniper berry, lavender, neroli, peppermint, rosemary, and tea tree? You may need to experiment with the ratio of carrier oil to solid ingredients to get a consistency you like.

Solid Deodorant

¼ cup cornstarch

¼ cup baking soda

¼ cup carrier oil or blend

¼–½ ounce beeswax

½–¾ teaspoon essential oil or blend

Combine the dry ingredients and set aside. Place the carrier oil and beeswax in a jar in a saucepan of water over low heat. Stir until the beeswax melts, then remove from heat. Let it cool before stirring in the essential oil. Using a fork, combine it with the dry ingredients and mix thoroughly. Store in a jar with a tight-fitting lid.

This type of deodorant is applied with the fingertips. As with any product used on your underarms, avoid applying it for at least half an hour after shaving. For best results with a spray deodorant, use a bottle with a fine mist setting.

Body Spray Deodorant

6 ounces water

1 ounce witch hazel

¼ teaspoon carrier oil or blend

¼ teaspoon essential oil or blend

Place the water and witch hazel in a bottle. Combine the carrier and essential oils and add them to the mixture. Shake well before each use.

• • • • • • •

Table 10.3 Essential Oils for Deodorants

Deodorant
Bergamot, cardamom, clary sage, coriander, cypress, eucalyptus, geranium, lavender, lemon, lemongrass, manuka, neroli, patchouli, peppermint, petitgrain, pine, ravintsara, sage, sandalwood, spearmint, tea tree, thyme, vetiver
Excessive Perspiration
Citronella, cypress, lemongrass, petitgrain, pine, sage

Many of the recipes detailed in this chapter can do double duty aromatically to support our emotions and general well-being, which we will explore in the next chapter.

CHAPTER 11

✦

Aromatherapy and Well-Being

The sense of smell is intimately linked with memory and emotion. This is because the olfactory cortex of the brain is an area closely tied to the limbic (emotional/visceral) system. There are thousands of olfactory receptors in a small area at the top of each nasal cavity. As we inhale, air passes over these receptors and information is carried along a nerve into the brain. In addition to transporting information, our sense of smell influences the functioning of the central nervous system.

Essential oils provide immediate access to the brain's rich storehouse of memory and emotion, which is why aromatherapy is a powerful treatment and enhancement for the emotions. Essential oils can help reduce stress and calm anxiety because inhaling scent affects the brain's activity. Scent can help us deal with a range of emotions, alter moods, and focus attention. Scent also enhances the ambience of a room, making it feel relaxed, energized, uplifted, or romantic.

Diffusing Essential Oils

The easiest way to use essential oils to support well-being is to diffuse them into the air. The various types of diffusers were covered in chapter 8. Even with newer gadgets on the market, the low-tech tealight diffuser is as popular as ever. In addition to the scent it releases, the flicker of candlelight is relaxing and soothing.

In the Middle Ages, bunches of aromatic herbs were hung throughout the house during the summer so the oxidizing essential oils could cool and refresh rooms. In the sixteenth century, violet, rosemary, and other distilled herbal waters were sprinkled on wooden floors to scent and cool rooms. A modern alternative is to sprinkle a couple of ribbons with an essential oil or blend and hang them in front of an open window or attach them to the front of a fan. In addition to dispersing scent throughout a room, oils such as mint can help cool a room. Using oils that repel

• • • • • • • •

insects can help keep pests away. Instead of sprinkling herbal water on the floor, as people did in the past, use a room spray. A bottle that has a fine mist spray is a low-tech version of a nebulizer.

Aromatherapy Room Spray

¼ cup vodka, unflavored

¼ teaspoon essential oil or blend

¼ cup water

Mix the vodka and essential oil in a spray bottle, then add the water. Shake well to mix and spray into the air.

Vodka in the room spray recipe acts as an emulsifier, holding together two things that do not combine: oil and water. Unflavored vodka is best because it does not usually have additives. The spray should not be stored, because over time, the alcohol in the vodka will interact with the essential oil and change the scent. Isopropyl alcohol, also known as rubbing alcohol, should never be used in a room spray because it is dangerous to ingest.

The Reed Diffuser

This off-the-grid method takes a little longer to disperse essential oil into the air, but it is a gentle and safe method.

Items needed to make a reed diffuser:

- A decorative glass or porcelain container
- Reeds
- Carrier oil
- Essential oil(s)

A short glass or porcelain jar or a vase with a narrow neck work best. Do not use a plastic container, because chemicals from the plastic can leach into the oils. A wide-mouth jar with a cork can be adjusted by drilling a hole in the cork so it is large enough to accommodate the reeds. There are several types of reeds on the market; however, rattan reeds work best, as they are porous and wick the oils more evenly. Reeds should be at least twice the height of the jar.

A lightweight carrier oil works best for the base oil because it is drawn up through the reeds more easily than a thick oil. While sweet almond is often recommended for the base, I have found that sunflower, being a thin oil, works best. If you are using more than one essential oil, blend them together first and allow about a week for the combined fragrance to mature.

Pour ¼ cup of carrier oil into your diffuser jar, add 2 teaspoons of essential oil or blend, and swirl to mix. Place the reeds in the jar. Turn the reeds upside down a couple of times the first day or two to get them started. After that, turn them once a day or every other day to disperse the scent. Over time, you will need to add more oil to the jar. When the reeds become completely saturated, replace them.

There are several things to avoid when making a reed diffuser. First, the fragrance oils on the market for reed diffusers are often synthetic and not essential oils. Some of them may smell nice, but they are made from chemicals. The commercial base oils for reed diffusers are often chemical-based too. Mineral oil and dipropylene glycol are sometimes recommended for a base oil, but avoid these for the same reason.

Other Methods of Aromatherapy

A warm bath is relaxing, but with essential oils it's even better. Place 12 to 18 drops of essential oil in an ounce of carrier oil to add to your bath. The carrier oil provides an even distribution of the essential oil. If you are a shower person, you can still take advantage of essential oils. Place 40 to 60 drops of essential oil on a washcloth. Fold it in half twice and place it on the floor of the shower under the water stream. An alternative to using a washcloth is to make shower melts.

When using shower melts, take care that the oil doesn't make the floor of the shower slippery. Depending on the temperature of your home or the time of year, you may need to store the shower melts in the refrigerator to keep them in a solid form. To use, place one on the floor of the shower. Use a washcloth or shower melts with stimulating scents when you need a pick-me-up.

Shower Melts

4 tablespoons cocoa butter or shea butter

1 tablespoon carrier oil or blend

40–60 drops essential oil or blend

Boil a little water in a saucepan and remove it from the heat. Place the cocoa or shea butter and the carrier oil in a jar in the water. Stir until the butter melts. Let it cool to room temperature, then add the essential oils. Pour the mixture into mini cupcake liners, then place them in the refrigerator for five or six hours. Let the mixture come to room temperature before storing.

When making recipes with cocoa or shea butter, the butter and carrier oil are usually heated twice to disperse any tiny clumps or particles that may form after the first heating. This is important for preparations used directly on the skin, but for shower melts, a smooth texture is not essential.

· · · · · · · ·

The easy vapors method (from chapter 8) used for respiratory issues also works nicely before bedtime to help relax and unwind. Boil a cup of water and pour it into a mug. Add 1 or 2 drops of essential oil, then hold the mug near your face to inhale the vapors.

Another method for relaxing and enhancing sleep is to sprinkle a few drops of essential oil on your pillow and/or sheets. Alternatively, place a reed diffuser by your bedside or sprinkle a few drops of essential oil on a cotton ball and tuck it into an organza bag to hang on a bedpost or place beside your pillow.

Massage is another way to deliver scent to your personal space. Mix 2 or 3 drops of essential oil in a teaspoon of carrier oil to massage your neck and temples. Rub a little into the pressure points on your wrists or the backs of your knees and let the warmth of your body activate the scent and waft the fragrance upward.

Aromatherapy on the Go

Aromatherapy is not limited to the home. Tuck an inhaler in your pocket or purse to take along wherever you go. At work or in a public place, waft a little scent under your nose as needed. If you are going to be driving or operating any type of equipment, avoid using very relaxing essential oils. Instead of reaching for an afternoon coffee, use peppermint in an inhaler to make you feel more alert.

In addition to being helpful when you have a cold, the nasal inhaler helps to deliver emotional support no matter where you are. In a pinch, place 2 to 3 drops of essential oil on a tissue, then tuck it into a plastic sandwich bag to take along.

Another way to enjoy aromatherapy on the go is to wear a diffuser locket, pendant, or bracelet. Aromatherapy beads are also available. These absorbent beads can be strung together into a necklace or bracelet. A few drops of essential oil can be applied before heading out of the house. In addition, a string of beads can be used like the traditional mala meditation beads, or make your own scented rosary beads for prayer.

Essential Oils for Emotional Support

As with perfumes and remedies, essential oils can be used singly or blended. Table 11.1 lists oils that can be used for emotional support. Good for general support, these oils are especially helpful if you just feel out of sorts. You may notice that a few, such as lavender, are listed for almost everything.

· · · · · · · ·

Table 11.1 Essential Oils for Emotional Support

Emotional Balance

Amyris, angelica, anise seed, basil, bay laurel, bergamot, cajeput, caraway seed, cardamom, carrot seed, cedarwood, celery seed, chamomile, cinnamon leaf, clary sage, coriander, cypress, elemi, eucalyptus (lemon), fennel, fir needle, frankincense, grapefruit, helichrysum, lavender, lemon, lime, mandarin, manuka, marjoram, myrrh, neroli, niaouli, patchouli, peppermint, petitgrain, pine, rosemary, sage, sandalwood, tea tree, thyme, vetiver, ylang-ylang

Focus and Mental Clarity

Amyris, basil, bay laurel, bergamot, black pepper, cajeput, cardamom, cedarwood, cinnamon leaf, citronella, clary sage, cypress, elemi, eucalyptus (lemon), frankincense, geranium, grapefruit, helichrysum, lavender, lemon, lemon balm, lemongrass, manuka, myrrh, neroli, niaouli, orange, palmarosa, patchouli, peppermint, petitgrain, pine, ravintsara, rosemary, sage, spearmint, tea tree

Grief; Dealing with Loss

Angelica, basil, bergamot, cedarwood, cypress, eucalyptus (blue), fir needle, geranium, lavender, lemon balm, marjoram, myrrh, patchouli, ravintsara, rose, rosemary, sandalwood, thyme, yarrow

Mental Fatigue

Angelica, basil, cajeput, caraway seed, cardamom, citronella, elemi, fir needle, ginger, hyssop, lemon, lime, mandarin, niaouli, palmarosa, peppermint, pine, ravintsara, rosemary, spearmint

Nervous Exhaustion

Bergamot, cinnamon leaf, coriander, elemi, ginger, grapefruit, helichrysum, lemongrass, manuka, palmarosa, patchouli, petitgrain, pine, ravintsara, rosemary, sage, vetiver

Nervous Tension

Angelica, basil, bergamot, cardamom, cedarwood, chamomile, clary sage, cypress, elemi, fir needle, frankincense, geranium, grapefruit, hyssop, juniper berry, lavender, lemon balm, mandarin, marjoram, neroli, orange, palmarosa, petitgrain, pine, ravintsara, rose, sage, spearmint, vetiver, ylang-ylang

Peace

Amyris, angelica, basil, bay laurel, bergamot, cedarwood, chamomile, clary sage, coriander, cypress, fir needle, geranium, ginger, helichrysum, lavender, lemon balm, marjoram, myrrh, neroli, orange, palmarosa, patchouli, pine, rose, sandalwood, ylang-ylang

Well-Being

Anise seed, bergamot, caraway seed, clove bud, coriander, eucalyptus, geranium, ginger, grapefruit, juniper berry, lavender, lemon, lime, mandarin, manuka, marjoram, myrrh, neroli, orange, petitgrain, pine, rose, ravintsara, rosemary, sandalwood, thyme

· · · · · · · ·

In the next chapter, we will explore the chakra system and how these energy centers are associated with various aspects of life. We will see how essential oils can be used to activate and move chakra energy.

.

CHAPTER 12

The Chakras and Well-Being

While the earliest known mention of the chakras appears in an ancient Hindu text called the *Vedas* (1500–800 BCE), it is generally accepted that knowledge of them dates to an earlier time.[11] According to the ancient texts, humans exist on a physical level as well as a subtle level, which encompasses the breath, the mind, feelings, and the ego. Chakras are energy fields in the subtle body, with corresponding energy centers in the nerve plexuses of the physical body. Seven of these nerve plexuses/energy centers constitute the major chakras that run from the base of the spine to the top of the head. Secondary chakras are located on the palms of the hands and soles of the feet.

The first three lower chakras are self-oriented and form the basis of our instincts about survival, sexuality, and courage. When we add the fourth chakra, the heart, our energy begins to move out of these basic needs and into the world. The fourth chakra acts as a fulcrum, balancing the three lower chakras, our foundation, with the three higher chakras, which are centered on expression, intuition, and spirituality.

Implying movement, the word *chakra* comes from Sanskrit, meaning "wheel," "center," or "spinning disc."[12] As such, their function is to keep energy moving. As energy spins within each chakra, it also sends energy to neighboring chakras, creating a flow of energy up and down the line of major chakras and throughout the entire body.

If energy stops flowing, it can become stuck in a chakra and cause issues that reverberate through related aspects of our lives. Using scent is an effective way to activate the energy of each

11. Chandra, *India Condensed*, 7.

12. Lowitz and Datta, *Sacred Sanskrit Words*, 65.

chakra and move it outward. By moving energy through the chakras, we can bring them into alignment and foster balance in our lives.

First Chakra: Root

The first chakra, or root chakra, is located at the base of the spine. It is our foundation and tap-root; it keeps us grounded. This chakra is concerned with survival, subsistence, and security. It is the seat of our fears, and if our energy gets stuck here, we live in fear. Activating and moving the energy of this chakra up through the others gives us a stable foundation upon which to build our lives. The color associated with the first chakra is red.

Second Chakra: Sacral

Located about an inch below the navel, the second chakra, or sacral chakra, is the seat of emotions. It is concerned with creation, procreation, and passion. It is about sensuality, sexuality, and balancing our needs and desires. It gives us the capacity to feel both pleasure and pain. If our energy gets stuck here, we can become emotionally unstable and easily addicted to things. Activating and moving this energy stokes our creativity and feeds our passions. It also helps us maintain healthy relationships. The color associated with the second chakra is orange.

Third Chakra: Solar Plexus

Located at the stomach, the third chakra, or solar plexus chakra, is our center of power and control. The experience it brings is strength and courage. It is the seat of our will. From this chakra, we are self-empowered. If our energy gets stuck here, we can become overpowering to others. Activating and moving this energy brings a healthy expression of confidence, authority, and leadership. The color associated with the third chakra is yellow.

Fourth Chakra: Heart

Located at the heart, the fourth chakra, or heart chakra, is our place of love and compassion. It is concerned with acceptance, trust, and relationships. From this chakra, we can be free from expectations and judgment. If our energy becomes stuck here, we lose touch with others; we react rather than respond to people and situations. Activating and moving this energy allows us to share our love and compassion with others and, equally important, feel these for ourselves. The color associated with the fourth chakra is green.

Fifth Chakra: Throat

The fifth chakra, or throat chakra, is our means for communicating with the world. It is concerned with our ability to share our inner world with others and to ask for what we want. This chakra relates to the second chakra and is our outlet for self-expression. When our energy is

. . . .

stuck here, we feel frustration and exhaustion. Activating and moving this energy allows us to take part in our community and share our gifts. The color associated with the fifth chakra is light blue.

Sixth Chakra: Third Eye

Located above and between the eyebrows, the sixth chakra, or third eye chakra, is the seat of awareness and intuition. This chakra brings insight and imagination. It helps us to be objective about ourselves and everything around us. When our energy gets stuck here, we are prevented from moving deeper into the self. Activating and moving this energy awakens our intuition, allowing us to "see" with more than our physical eyes. The color associated with the sixth chakra is indigo blue.

Seventh Chakra: Crown

The seventh chakra, or crown chakra, is located on the top of the head and is the seat of spirituality and our connection with cosmic consciousness and universal energy. It brings understanding and a sense of being. It helps us find our place in the web of life. If our energy is stuck here, we are unable to focus and we are thrown off the path we want to follow. Activating and moving this energy brings peace and a deep connection with spirituality. The colors associated with the seventh chakra are white and violet.

Table 12.1 Essential Oils and the Chakras

The First (or Root) Chakra
Angelica (root), carrot seed, cedarwood, celery seed, chamomile, clove bud, elemi, fir needle, frankincense, ginger, lavender, lemongrass, myrrh, niaouli, patchouli, rose, rosemary, sandalwood, thyme, vetiver
The Second (or Sacral) Chakra
Amyris, anise seed, bergamot, cajeput, caraway seed, cardamom, carrot seed, cedarwood, chamomile, citronella, clary sage, coriander, fennel, fir needle, frankincense, ginger, helichrysum, hyssop, juniper berry, lavender, lemon balm, manuka, neroli, niaouli, orange, patchouli, ravintsara, rose, sandalwood, tea tree, ylang-ylang
The Third (or Solar Plexus) Chakra
Basil, bay laurel, black pepper, cardamom, cedarwood, chamomile, cinnamon leaf, clove bud, coriander, cypress, frankincense, geranium, ginger, grapefruit, hyssop, juniper berry, lavender, lemon, lemongrass, mandarin, manuka, niaouli, patchouli, peppermint, petitgrain, ravintsara, rose, rosemary, sandalwood, spearmint, tea tree, vetiver, ylang-ylang

Table 12.1 Essential Oils and the Chakras (*continued*)

The Fourth (or Heart) Chakra
Anise seed, bergamot, caraway seed, cardamom, cedarwood, chamomile, cinnamon leaf, citronella, coriander, cypress, eucalyptus, frankincense, geranium, ginger, lavender, lemon, lemon balm, lime, mandarin, manuka, marjoram, neroli, niaouli, orange, palmarosa, patchouli, pine, ravintsara, rose, sandalwood, tea tree, vetiver, ylang-ylang
The Fifth (or Throat) Chakra
Amyris, basil, bergamot, cajeput, caraway seed, cedarwood, chamomile, citronella, clary sage, cypress, fennel, fir needle, frankincense, geranium, grapefruit, hyssop, lavender, lemongrass, lime, mandarin, myrrh, niaouli, orange, palmarosa, patchouli, peppermint, petitgrain, pine, ravintsara, rose, rosemary, sage, sandalwood, spearmint, thyme, vetiver
The Sixth (or Third Eye) Chakra
Angelica (seed), anise seed, bay laurel, black pepper, cajeput, cedarwood, chamomile, cinnamon leaf, clary sage, cypress, elemi, frankincense, helichrysum, juniper berry, lavender, lemon, marjoram, myrrh, patchouli, peppermint, petitgrain, pine, rose, rosemary, sandalwood, spearmint, thyme, vetiver
The Seventh (or Crown) Chakra
Angelica (seed), cedarwood, chamomile, clary sage, elemi, fir needle, frankincense, geranium, helichrysum, lavender, myrrh, neroli, palmarosa, patchouli, rose, sage, sandalwood, vetiver

How to Work with the Chakras

As you may have noticed in table 12.1, some essential oils, such as frankincense and lavender, are listed for all the chakras. These oils can be used to work with an individual chakra or to bring all seven chakras into balance.

A single essential oil or a blend of oils can be used when working with chakra energy. The oil can be applied to the body at the location of the chakra. For most of the chakras, you can mix the essential oil with a carrier oil at a 2% dilution (see table 8.1). For the throat and third eye chakras, use a 1% dilution. Take a moment to smell the fragrance of the oil, then dab a tiny bit of it on the area of the chakra.

Instead of applying an essential oil to the body, a few drops can be placed in the melted wax of a pillar candle. Let it burn for several minutes to disperse the scent before doing the following chakra-balancing exercise. To boost the effectiveness of the candle, coordinate its color with the color associated with a chakra. If you are working with tealight candles, coordinate the color of the candleholder with the chakra. Multiple oils and/or candles can be used when working with more than one chakra. A diffuser can also be used, but make sure any noise it makes will not disturb you.

• • • • • • •

As with meditation or any spiritual practice, find a time to perform this chakra-balancing exercise when you will not be rushed or interrupted. Decide which chakra you want to work with, then apply the oil, light a candle, or start a diffuser. Close your eyes and focus on the scent for a moment or two, then mindfully think about the aspects and attributes of the chakra. Briefly think about what may cause you to feel at odds with them.

Begin the process of bringing the chakra into balance with the energy of the others. Focus your attention on the root chakra and visualize it spinning. Imagine the energy as soft white light that slowly moves up to the second chakra. Visualize that one spinning too.

Work your way up through all seven chakras. Feel the energy moving through you, up your spine, and then around you. Visualize being surrounded by white light. Once you have done this, let the image slowly fade from your mind. Sit for a few minutes and focus your attention on the floor and your connection with Mother Earth. Spend a few minutes sitting quietly, and when you feel ready, return to your normal activities.

When going through this exercise, it may take longer to visualize the problem chakra spinning, or it may not spin the first time you try it. If a chakra does not spin, go on to the next one. Even if you cannot visualize or sense a chakra spinning, the energy of the other chakras moving around it will help break the inertia. You may have to go through the exercise a few times to accomplish this. After all, chakra energy doesn't suddenly become stuck, so getting it unstuck also takes time. With patience and gentle work, you can get the energy flowing.

While this exercise is useful for dealing with problems, it can be used even if you just feel out of sorts. It is also helpful before meditation to balance your energy. To further our work with energy, we will move on to spirituality and candle magic in the next chapter.

CHAPTER 13

Spiritual and Magical Uses of Essential Oils

Scents have been an integral part of spiritual practices in many religions. In addition to memories and emotions, scents can help us find the deeper parts of ourselves that reach into our souls. Derived from the Latin word *esse*, meaning "to be," the word *essence* can refer to the intrinsic nature of something or an extract from a plant; spirit or fragrance.[13] Whether we're sending out healing prayers or magical intentions, essential oils can help us tap into the wellspring of energy we carry within.

Scent and Spirituality

Fragrance can help us communicate with our deeper self and connect with our spirituality. Burning a candle lends support to spiritual practices by energetically clearing and enhancing the energy of an area. This is especially helpful around an altar or a special place for meditation or prayer. The candle can be one that you made, or you can add a few drops of essential oil to the pool of melted wax in a pillar candle. Frankincense, lavender, and sandalwood are especially potent for any form of spiritual practice.

Just as ancient people used scents as offerings to give thanks to their deities, we can too. Tealight candles work well as votives, and when you make your own (which we will cover later in this chapter), they can support your specific purpose. Refer to table 13.1 for oils that correspond with certain purposes. Reed diffusers also work nicely to enhance spiritual practices and

---

13. *Oxford Dictionary of English*, s.v. "essence," 598.

observances. As an alternative, dab an essential oil or blend (diluted, of course) on your wrists; this is especially effective for prayer and meditation.

When consecrating an altar or clearing the energy of a space to be used for meditation, prayer, or ritual, waft the scent above and below the altar and around the entire area. A candle or tealight diffuser can also be used for sending forth prayers. As an offering to express gratitude, use a small bowl or cup and place a few drops of essential oil or blend in it as you speak or think about your reason for feeling grateful. Do the same thing when calling on help from angels or other special beings.

As mentioned in chapter 11, aromatherapy beads can be strung together to make meditation or rosary beads. Apply a few drops of essential oil to the beads and let dry. The heat of your hands will activate the scent while you meditate or pray.

Table 13.1 Essential Oils for Spiritual Support

Consecrate an Altar or Clear the Energy of a Space
Angelica, anise seed, basil, bay laurel, black pepper, cedarwood, cinnamon leaf, coriander, cypress, fennel, frankincense, geranium, helichrysum, hyssop, lavender, lime, manuka, myrrh, palmarosa, patchouli, pine, ravintsara, rose, rosemary, sandalwood, tea tree, thyme
General Support for Meditation and Spiritual Practices
Amyris, angelica, bay laurel, bergamot, cinnamon leaf, clary sage, clove bud, elemi, fir needle, frankincense, geranium, grapefruit, helichrysum, hyssop, juniper berry, lavender, lemon, lemon balm, mandarin, myrrh, niaouli, palmarosa, patchouli, pine, ravintsara, rose, sage, sandalwood, spearmint, vetiver, ylang-ylang
Grounding and Centering for Meditation or Prayer
Angelica, black pepper, cajeput, cardamom, citronella, cypress, elemi, fir needle, ginger, helichrysum, juniper berry, lavender, lemongrass, manuka, marjoram, myrrh, palmarosa, patchouli, pine, ravintsara, sage, sandalwood, thyme, vetiver
Express Gratitude
Frankincense, myrrh, sage
Healing Prayers
Angelica, basil, bay laurel, black pepper, cajeput, cardamom, carrot seed, chamomile, coriander, elemi, eucalyptus, fennel, fir needle, frankincense, geranium, lavender, manuka, myrrh, niaouli, palmarosa, peppermint, rose, sage, sandalwood, thyme
Special Help and Calling on Angels
Angelica, basil, frankincense, myrrh, rose, sandalwood

• • • • • • • •

How to Make Scented Candles

Making tealight candles is quick and easy enough to do for a specific purpose, such as sending healing prayers. Tealight cups are available at most craft stores and online. For larger candles, Mason jars and decorative glass or metal containers can be used. Be sure they are safe enough to hold hot liquid. In addition to spiritual practices, scented candles are great for aromatherapy, feng shui, and, of course, candle magic.

Items needed for making candles:

- Tealight cups or a Mason jar
- A glass measuring cup
- Saucepan large enough to hold the measuring cup or jar
- Knife for stirring
- Wax
- Coconut oil (when using beeswax)
- Essential oil or blend
- Carrier oil to give the scent staying power
- Wicks
- Clip-style clothespins, pencils, or hairpins (optional)

The base ingredient for candles is, of course, wax, and there are three popular types: paraffin, soy, and beeswax. Paraffin is a petroleum byproduct and not a great choice for aromatherapy and other practices for well-being.

Soy wax is easy to work with and clean up; however, a point to consider is that almost all the soybean crop is genetically modified and may contain pesticides. During my research, I was unable to find a source that could guarantee non-GMO soy wax. The term *pure* or *100% pure* on the label means only that it was not mixed with any other type of wax, such as paraffin.

Beeswax is the oldest material used to make candles and produces less smoke than other waxes. While it is more expensive, it is a natural product that is especially good if you have allergies. Like soy, it can be mixed with other waxes, so look for 100% pure beeswax. On its own, it has a light, sweet scent that does not usually interfere with essential oil fragrances. For more about beeswax, refer to part 7.

Soy wax is sold in blocks and flakes, and beeswax in blocks and pellets, also called *pastilles* or *beads*. Blocks of wax can be grated like cheese, which makes it easy to measure and melt. Beeswax is also sold in convenient one-ounce bars. To measure smaller amounts, cut the bar in half (for ½ ounce) or in half again, if necessary. Because beeswax is hard, place a bar in a plastic bag and set it in a bowl of hot tap water for about ten to fifteen minutes to soften and make it easier to cut.

Wicks have small metal tabs at one end that go in the bottom of the jar or cup. While tealight candles are easy to work with, keeping a wick centered in a jar for a larger candle can be a little tricky. To help, place a clip-style clothespin on its side across the top of the jar and thread the wick up through the spring. Wrapping the top of the wick around a pencil or barbeque skewer also works to keep it in place. If you are using beeswax, another way to keep the wick in place is to dip the tab in the melted wax and stick it to the bottom of the container.

The amount of wax and essential oil used in the following recipes is a basic guideline and depends on the type of wax used. When using beeswax, mix approximately 3 parts beeswax to 1 part coconut oil, which will help it solidify more evenly. When using a blend of essential oils, mix them together first so you can adjust the balance of scents. The amount of essential oil or blend depends on the strength of the oils you use.

The tealight cups that I use are ½ inch deep and 1½ inches wide. As an alternative, use a mini cupcake pan for your candle molds. As with blending essential oils and making remedies, take notes while making candles so you will know how you might want to adjust the amounts of oils and wax the next time.

For an 8-Ounce Jar Candle

5 ounces wax

3 tablespoons coconut oil (if using beeswax)

3–4 teaspoons essential oil or blend

For 3–4 Tealight Candles

1 ounce wax

2 teaspoons coconut oil (if using beeswax)

1–2 teaspoons essential oil or blend

Place a glass measuring cup with the wax and coconut oil in a saucepan of water and warm over low heat. Stir continuously until the wax melts, then remove it from the heat. If you are using beeswax, when it has melted, dip the bottom of the wick tab in the wax and set it in the bottom of the jar or tealight cup.

Allow the mixture to cool slightly. While it is still liquid, mix in the essential oil. You may need to set the measuring cup in the pan of hot water for a minute if the essential oil congeals in the wax. Pour the wax into the jar or tealight cups, but keep a little aside. As the wax cools, it may sink slightly in the middle around the wick. It may also crack or pull away from the sides of the container. Warm the leftover wax and add it to the jar or tealight cup to fill in these spaces. When the wax is cool, trim the wicks and give the candles a couple of days to set before using.

• • • • • • • •

Candle Magic

Because fire is regarded as the element of transformation, candles are an important component for ritual and spells. In fact, candle magic is often used as an introduction to magic and spell casting. Aromatic oils have been used since ancient times for a range of purposes, including magic. Carrying the life essence of plants, essential oils are considered particularly potent to help focus thought, support willpower, and carry forth magical intent.

Engaging the mind through visualization is an important component of magic work. Visualization is the use of mental images that run like a cinema in our mind. Daydreams are an example of this; however, in magic it is important to stay for the whole film. In daydreams we may flit back and forth between the images in our mind and the outside world, but visualization in magic requires focus. It is also important to be specific and realistic about what you want to achieve as you visualize the outcome.

There are two ways that essential oils can be used in candle magic. One is to consecrate or prepare a candle with oil, and the second is to make a candle. If you are using essential oil to prepare a candle, you will need a new unused one. Because the candle needs to burn completely down in spell work, it's best to use a small one. The type of candle called a *tiny taper*, which is very thin and only about five inches tall, works well. If you make your own, make a tealight for candle magic. The advantage of making your own candle is that you can begin the magical process by focusing your mind on your purpose while you are stirring and pouring the wax.

If you are consecrating a candle that you purchased, put a small amount of essential oil or blend on your fingertip and draw a line from the base of the candle to the top. Repeat this on the other side of the candle. Going from bottom to top aids in directing your energy and willpower outward. If it is for banishing or grounding purposes, draw lines with the oil from the top to the bottom of the candle. This will pull energy and negativity down to the ground, where it will be neutralized.

When you are ready for magic, place your candle on a table or meditation altar where you can sit comfortably in front of it. Close your eyes for a moment and think about your purpose. When you are ready, light the candle and whisper:

Now is the time to begin;
may this purpose I soon win.
By this candle burning bright,
work my magic on this night.

Visualize all the steps that you would need to take to accomplish your purpose or reach your goal. Engage all of your senses as you visualize how you will feel at the outcome. Be aware of energy building inside you as you experience achieving your goal. Open your eyes and gaze at the candle. Visualize the energy you feel merging with the candle flame and growing. Sometimes it helps to imagine energy as a soft white or golden light. When you feel the energy increasing and reaching a crescendo, visualize that you are releasing it out to the world. Afterward, empty your mind of thoughts, then slowly bring your attention to your feet on the floor and your energy connecting with the earth and keeping you grounded. Sit in silence as you watch the candle burn out.

Table 13.2 Essential Oils for Magic

Abundance and Prosperity Basil, bay laurel, carrot seed, cedarwood, chamomile, fir needle, ginger, grapefruit, helichrysum, juniper berry, lemon, lime, mandarin, manuka, myrrh, orange, peppermint, pine, sage, vetiver
Banish and Remove Negativity Amyris, angelica, anise seed, basil, black pepper, cardamom, cedarwood, citronella, clove bud, cypress, elemi, eucalyptus (lemon), frankincense, hyssop, juniper berry, manuka, niaouli, palmarosa, patchouli, peppermint, pine, ravintsara, rosemary, sage, sandalwood, tea tree
Happiness Anise seed, basil, clary sage, clove bud, cypress, eucalyptus (blue), fir needle, frankincense, geranium, juniper berry, lemon, lemon balm, mandarin, marjoram, neroli, orange, patchouli, ravintsara, rose, sandalwood, thyme, ylang-ylang
Justice Bay laurel, bergamot, black pepper, cedarwood, cinnamon leaf, cypress, frankincense, niaouli, patchouli, pine, sandalwood
Love Anise seed, basil, bergamot, cardamom, chamomile, coriander, fennel, frankincense, geranium, ginger, lavender, lemon balm, lime, marjoram, neroli, orange, palmarosa, patchouli, rose, rosemary, sandalwood, spearmint, thyme, vetiver, ylang-ylang
Luck Anise seed, bergamot, caraway seed, chamomile, cinnamon leaf, clove bud, geranium, lemongrass, patchouli, peppermint, rose, rosemary, sandalwood, spearmint, thyme, vetiver
Success Angelica, basil, bay laurel, bergamot, black pepper, cajeput, chamomile, cinnamon leaf, clove bud, frankincense, geranium, grapefruit, juniper berry, lemon, lemon balm, lime, mandarin, myrrh, orange, sandalwood

• • • • • • •

Essential oils and candles also provide support for other metaphysical practices. For these, you can light a candle to burn while engaging in these activities or dab an essential oil or blend on your wrists. For dream work, the latter method should be used for safety reasons. As an alternative, place a few drops of essential oil on a cotton ball and tuck it into a small organza bag. Hang the bag on a bedpost or place it next to your pillow.

Table 13.3 Essential Oils for Other Practices

Dream Work
Amyris, angelica, anise seed, bay laurel, bergamot, black pepper, caraway seed, cedarwood, chamomile, cinnamon leaf, clary sage, eucalyptus, frankincense, helichrysum, juniper berry, lavender, lemon balm, marjoram, orange, rose, rosemary, sandalwood, spearmint, vetiver
Past-Life Work
Amyris, eucalyptus, frankincense, lemon balm, myrrh, rosemary, sandalwood

In the next section, we move on to using essential oils in the home for cleaning and pest control. Also included is a chapter on aromatic feng shui, which we can use to change and enhance the energy of our home.

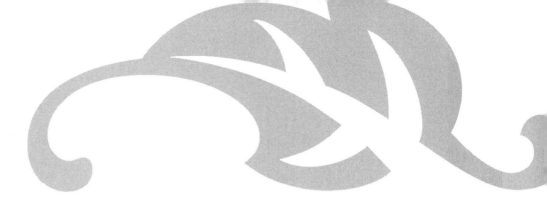

PART FIVE

Using Essential Oils in the Home

This section brings us to yet another aspect of essential oils, which is their application in the home. In addition to creating economical homemade products, we can also reduce or avoid the use of harmful chemicals in our homes. While most essential oils can be used to scent the air, some do more than make a room smell nice; they clean the air and remove stale odors.

Good old-fashioned cleaning supplies that have been used for decades can be given an update by adding essential oils. With bacteria-fighting properties, some oils can boost the effectiveness of homemade preparations. Most likely, you already have the base ingredients in your kitchen. If not, they are readily available in grocery stores.

In addition to providing basic recipes for house-cleaning products, this section includes important details on some of the base ingredients. We will discover what different types of vinegar do, what should not be mixed with vinegar, and what should not be used on certain surfaces in the home. Keep in mind that the information from part 2 on blending essential oils for scent can help you create cleaning products that are uniquely your own.

While nobody likes to have bugs lurking around their home, using commercial products that are filled with (often dangerous) chemicals is not comforting either. We will learn which essential oils repel which creepy-crawlies and how to use them. Some oils even deter rodents. Whether you are using essential oils for cleaning or pest control, be sure to do so carefully, especially if you have small children or pets.

If you have used feng shui or just thought about trying it, included is what I call *aromatic feng shui*. The final chapter provides a step-by-step guide for applying the basic principles of this ancient Chinese practice using essential oils to modify and enhance the energy of your home.

• • • • • • •

CHAPTER 14

⤳

Caring for the Home

Saving money is not the only reason to use homemade cleaning supplies; avoiding harmful chemicals is even more important. Along with the manual that came with my new stove was a sample packet of a cleaning product. I thought it was a nice idea until I noticed the skull and crossbones next the word *Danger*. A product with this kind of warning is not something I want to use in my house, much less in my kitchen, where I prepare food.

The "old-fashioned" cleaning supplies that my grandmother made are coming back in vogue and can be given an update by incorporating essential oils. With bacteria-fighting properties, many oils such as bergamot, eucalyptus, lavender, lemongrass, tea tree, and thyme can boost the effectiveness of cleaning preparations. Use the oils individually or blend a special scent to use in certain rooms or throughout your home. This can be especially nice during the winter holiday season.

Most likely you already have the base ingredients in your cupboard. If not, they can be picked up at the grocery store. If you have pets in your home, be sure to read the pet precautions in chapter 4.

Base Ingredients

Vinegar is excellent for cleaning, but there are a few things to know about it. White vinegar, sometimes called *spirit vinegar*, is more acidic and better for tough cleaning jobs. Distilled vinegar, sometimes called *distilled white vinegar*, is slightly milder but works well for general cleaning. Another type is called *cleaning vinegar*. This is even more acidic than white vinegar and is not suitable for cooking.

Sodium bicarbonate, or baking soda, is a mixture of sodium and hydrogen carbonate and is a mainstay of baking. It is well known as part of the dynamic duo of cleaning when combined

· · · · · · · ·

with vinegar. As an alkaline, it reacts with an acid, such as vinegar, and releases carbon dioxide gas. Bubbling baking soda can make a cake rise or clean a kitchen drain.

Used for cleaning since the Middle Ages, salt is a good scouring agent for hard surfaces; however, it should not be used on marble, linoleum, or waxed floors. Keep sea salt for cooking and beauty products and use plain table salt for cleaning.

Castile soap is a vegetable-based soap named for the Castile region of Spain, where olive oil–based soaps originated. Today, Castile soap is made with a blend of oils, usually coconut, sunflower, and castor. Castile soap is extremely alkaline. Unlike baking soda, which is mildly alkaline and makes a good combo with vinegar, Castile soap does not. Having opposite polarities on the pH scale, Castile soap and vinegar neutralize each other and result in a curdled yucky mess.

Table 14.1 Essential Oils for Freshening and Cleaning

Freshen and Deodorize
Angelica, anise seed, bay laurel, bergamot, cedarwood, citronella, clary sage, clove bud, fir needle, ginger, grapefruit, helichrysum, juniper berry, lavender, lemon, lemongrass, lime, mandarin, neroli, orange, palmarosa, patchouli, petitgrain, pine, ravintsara, sage, sandalwood, spearmint, tea tree, thyme
Surface Cleaning
Bergamot, cardamom, clove bud, grapefruit, helichrysum, lavender, lemon, lime, manuka, orange, palmarosa, pine, sandalwood, tea tree, thyme
Mold and Mildew
Cinnamon leaf, clove bud, eucalyptus, lavender, lemon, peppermint, rosemary, tea tree, thyme
Wood Furniture
Cedarwood, lavender, lemon, orange, pine

Freshen and Deodorize

While most essential oils can be used to scent the air, the ones listed in table 14.1 do more than make a room smell nice. They clean the air and remove stale odors. Use these oils in a diffuser in any area that needs help.

One simple thing that many of us do is put a box or cup of baking soda in the refrigerator to absorb odors and keep it smelling fresh. Adding a little essential oil to the baking soda also adds freshness. Depending on the oil(s) you choose, it can also help fight germs.

Fridge Freshener

8-ounce box of baking soda

4–6 drops essential oil or blend

Combine the ingredients and mix well, using a fork to break up clumps. Pour the mixture into a decorative container and place in the refrigerator.

The fridge freshener should be replaced every three months, but don't throw the old stuff in the garbage. Add a little more essential oil, then pour it in your kitchen sink drain to take away odors. Let it sit for a few minutes, then flush with hot water.

Carpet Powder

8 ounces baking soda

1/4 teaspoon essential oil or blend

Mix the ingredients thoroughly, using a fork to break up clumps. Lightly sprinkle the powder over a carpet. Let it sit for thirty minutes to an hour before vacuuming.

The room spray noted in chapter 11 for aromatherapy also works well to freshen upholstery. Do a patch test on the fabric first to ensure that the spray will not damage it. The vodka in the spray acts as an emulsifier to combine the water and essential oil. All three ingredients evaporate.

Upholstery or Room Spray

¼ cup water

¼ cup unflavored vodka

¼ teaspoon essential oil or blend

Mix the vodka and essential oil in a bottle with a fine mist spray nozzle. Add the water, shake, then spray lightly over upholstery and cushions or into the air.

A variation on the carpet powder can be used as an alternative to the room spray. Place a jar of the mixture in an out-of-the-way spot in the bathroom, laundry room, or other area prone to unpleasant odors.

Room Freshening Powder

8 ounces baking soda

½ teaspoon essential oil or blend

Mix the ingredients thoroughly, then pour into a decorative jar. Cover with cheesecloth and tie in place with a ribbon.

Chapter 14

General Cleaning

As with freshening the air, some essential oils not only smell good but also fight germs. A general-purpose surface cleaner for the kitchen and bath can be made in two ways: one with vinegar and the other with Castile soap. The vinegar surface cleaner should not be used on marble or granite because it can cause damage.

Vinegar Surface Cleaner

1 cup water

1 cup white vinegar

15 drops essential oil or blend

Combine all ingredients in a spray bottle and gently shake. Spray on the surface, then wipe off with a clean dry cloth.

Castile Soap Surface Cleaner

2 cups water

2–4 tablespoons Castile soap

15 drops essential oil or blend

Combine all ingredients in a spray bottle and gently shake. Spray on the surface, then wipe off with a damp cloth.

With fresh clean scents, citrus oils make good surface cleaners. They are also good for cleaning glass and do wonders in the dishwasher and microwave.

Glass Cleaner

1½ cups white vinegar

½ cup water

15 drops citrus essential oil or blend

Combine all ingredients in a spray bottle and shake well. Use on windows and mirrors as you would any other glass cleaner.

Dishwasher Cleaner

1 cup vinegar

6–8 drops essential oil

Place the ingredients in a bowl on the top rack of the dishwasher. Run the machine through a full cycle without any other dishes inside.

Microwave Cleaner

½ cup water

½ cup vinegar

2 drops essential oil

Combine ingredients in a microwave-safe mug or bowl. Place it in the microwave and run on high power for five or six minutes. Afterward, use the solution to wipe down the interior.

Essential oils also come to the rescue to fight mold and mildew The following recipe can be used as a bathtub and tile cleaner or to wipe out washers and dishwashers that smell musty. After removing mold and mildew, use the inhibitor spray on a regular basis as a preventive measure. Test a small area of tile first. Also, avoid using these recipes on marble or granite, as vinegar can damage these surfaces.

Mold and Mildew Remover

1 cup water

1 cup vinegar

½ teaspoon essential oil

Combine the ingredients in a spray bottle. Shake well and spray on the surface. Let it sit for a minute, then wipe off.

Mold and Mildew Inhibitor

¼ cup water

½ cup unflavored vodka

8–12 drops essential oil or blend

Combine the vodka and essential oil in a bottle with a fine mist spray. Add the water, shake well, and spray into the air in areas where mold and mildew are a problem.

The protective finish on wood furniture needs a boost from time to time to keep it looking good. Because changes in humidity can affect wood, making it expand or shrink, a nourishing polish can help prevent cracking and splitting. Test a small area of wood with the furniture polish first.

Furniture Polish

6–8 tablespoons olive oil

½ ounce beeswax

10–15 drops essential oil or blend

· · · · · · · ·

Place the olive oil and beeswax in a jar in a saucepan of water. Warm it over low heat, stirring until the beeswax melts. Let the mixture cool, then add the essential oil. Mix thoroughly.

Use a soft cloth to apply a thin layer of polish. Let it dry, then buff it with a clean dry cloth. Polish furniture every three to four months or as needed. After cleaning the house or working outdoors, there's nothing like a good scrub to clean and restore hard-working hands.

Hand Scrub

¼ cup coarse sea salt

¼ cup sugar (brown or white)

3 tablespoons coconut oil

½ teaspoon essential oil or blend

Combine the dry ingredients in a bowl. Melt the coconut oil, if necessary, and combine it with the essential oil. Stir the oils into the dry ingredients. Store the mixture in a jar with a tight-fitting lid.

Sugar is added to the scrub recipe to soften the abrasiveness of the salt. If you have sensitive skin, use only sugar without salt.

Laundry Room and Closets

Clean laundry starts with a clean washer. The following recipe deodorizes and dissolves soap residue in the washtub and pipes. Use it without clothes in the machine.

Wash the Washer

3–4 cups vinegar

½ cup baking soda

1 teaspoon essential oil or blend

Set the washer to the largest load setting and fill it with hot water. Pour in the vinegar, start the cycle, and let it agitate for a minute. Add the baking soda and essential oils and let it agitate again for a minute. Stop the washer and let it sit for up to an hour. While the washer is stopped, dip a cloth into the water and use it to wipe down the bleach and fabric softener dispensers and around the rim of the tub. Resume the wash cycle and let it finish.

To scent laundry, place 3 to 6 drops of essential oil or blend in a cup of water and pour it in the fabric softener dispenser. This is a nice way to scent linens. Scent can also be added to clothes when ironing.

• • • • • • • •

Ironing Spray

¼ cup water

5–7 drops essential oil or blend

Combine ingredients in a bottle with a fine mist spray nozzle. Lightly spray the ironing board before starting each piece of clothing or as needed.

Sachets can be hung in closets or placed in drawers to scent clothing and linens. The recipe in the next section is multifunctional for scenting and/or keeping pests at bay.

Natural Pest Control

While we generally don't like bugs in our homes, the chemicals in commercial products can be equally daunting. That said, essential oils should be used carefully, especially if you have small children and/or pets in the home.

Table 14.2 Essential Oils and Other Ingredients for Pest Control

Essential Oil	Repels
Basil laurel	Insects, especially earwigs, flies, mice, moths, roaches
Cajeput	Insects, especially fleas, lice, mosquitoes
Cardamom	Insects, especially ants, flies, moths
Cedarwood	Insects, especially fleas, mice, mosquitoes, moths, rats, ticks
Cinnamon leaf	Insects, especially ants, flies, lice, mosquitoes, roaches
Citronella	Insects, especially fleas, mice, mosquitoes, moths, rats, spiders
Clove bud	Insects, especially flies, mosquitoes, spiders
Cypress	Insects, especially moths, roaches
Eucalyptus (blue)	Insects, especially fleas, flies, gnats, lice, mosquitoes, moths, spiders
Eucalyptus (lemon)*	Insects, especially fleas, flies, gnats, mosquitoes, moths, roaches, silverfish, spiders
Geranium	Insects, especially fleas, lice, mosquitoes
Hyssop	Insects, especially flies, moths
Juniper berry	Insects, especially flies, mosquitoes
Lavender	Insects, especially ants, fleas, flies, lice, mosquitoes, moths, spiders
Lemon	Insects, especially gnats, mosquitoes, spiders
Lemon balm	Insects, especially mosquitoes
Lemongrass	Insects, especially fleas, gnats, lice, mosquitoes, ticks
Manuka	Insects, especially gnats, mosquitoes, spiders

· · · · · · · ·

Table 14.2 Essential Oils and Other Ingredients
for Pest Control (*continued*)

Essential Oil	Repels
Niaouli	Insects, especially mosquitoes, moths
Orange	Insects, especially ants, fleas, spiders, ticks
Palmarosa	Insects, especially fleas, mosquitoes
Patchouli	Insects, especially ants, gnats, mosquitoes, moths
Peppermint	Insects, especially ants, aphids, bees, fleas, flies, gnats, mice, mosquitoes, moths, rats, roaches, spiders
Pine	Insects, especially fleas, lice, moths
Ravintsara	Insects, especially flies, mosquitoes, moths, silverfish, spiders
Rosemary	Insects, especially caterpillars, flies, gnats, lice, mosquitoes
Spearmint	Insects, especially ants, aphids, fleas, gnats, mice
Tea tree	Insects, especially ants, fleas, flies, gnats, lice, mosquitoes, moths, silverfish, spiders
Thyme	Insects, especially chiggers, flies, lice, mosquitoes, roaches, ticks
Vetiver	Insects, especially mosquitoes, moths
Other Ingredients	**Repels**
Shea butter	Insects, especially mosquitoes
Vinegar	Insects, especially ants, fruit flies, spiders

*Lemon eucalyptus is the only essential oil on the EPA (Environmental Protection Agency) list of registered insect repellents for mosquitoes.[14]

A sachet is effective to freshen a linen closet or protect winter clothes when you put them away for the summer. The following recipe contains enough for several 3 x 5-inch muslin bags. When the scent fades, refresh the sachets with a few drops of essential oil.

Pest Control Sachets
30–40 drops essential oil or blend

1 teaspoon carrier oil

1 cup baking soda

Combine the essential oils with the carrier oil. Stir in the baking soda and mix thoroughly with a fork to break up any lumps. Let the mixture dry, then pour into muslin bags.

14. Centers for Disease Control and Prevention, list of insect repellents for mosquitoes, https://www.cdc.gov/zika/prevention/prevent-mosquito-bites.html.

If you can find where creepy-crawlies enter your home, spraying the area can work as a deterrent. As an alternative, liberally sprinkle a few cotton balls with essential oil to tuck into out-of-the-way nooks and crannies or cupboards.

Keep Bugs Out Spray

¼ cup white vinegar

¼ cup water

½ teaspoon essential oil or blend

Combine all the ingredients in a spray bottle. Shake well before each use.

Diffusers and candles can also be used to discourage insects. Patio luminaries provide a festive and decorative touch for a pest-free outdoor zone.

Patio Luminaire

2 or 3 herb sprigs: basil, lavender, and/or rosemary

½ teaspoon essential oil or blend

18-ounce Mason jar

5–6 ounces water

1 tealight candle

Place the herbs and essential oil in the jar, then add the water. Carefully add the tealight candle so it floats on top of the water.

Now that we have seen how essential oils can be used to freshen and clean, in the next chapter we will explore the ancient art of feng shui to work with and adjust the energy of the home.

CHAPTER 15

⟡

Balance Energy in the Home with Aromatic Feng Shui

Although this ancient Chinese practice can be complicated, by working with its basic principles of yin and yang, we can use essential oils to apply the concepts of feng shui and get results. The most fundamental principle of feng shui—creating flow, harmony, and balance—is about balancing energy and maintaining harmony in one's environment. This concept is often illustrated with the yin-yang symbol.

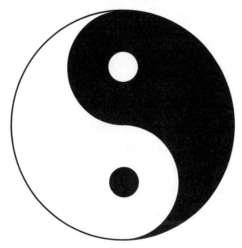

Figure 15.1 The Yin-Yang Symbol Illustrates the Basic Principle of Feng Shui of Creating Flow, Harmony, and Balance

Although the light and dark sections of the yin-yang symbol are equal, they do not split the circle in half down the middle; instead, they flow into each other. This symbol illustrates not only that each is necessary to create a whole but also that each contains a little of the other. Just as the sunlight of day is necessary for growth, the cool quiet of night is necessary for rest.

Yin and yang can best be described as a harmonious dynamic of opposites. They are regarded as the binding forces that hold the universe together and are present in all things. Because the forces of yin and yang are constantly changing, the universe is anything but static. As anyone who has done any type of energy work knows, it is an ongoing process. Maintaining a healthy environment takes a little awareness about how energy flows.

According to feng shui, negative energy is called *sha*, and it occurs where yin and yang are out of balance. Sha can occur in two extremes: it can be fast-moving (too yang) or stagnating and depleted (too yin). In the home, when energy is trapped in a corner of a room, it stagnates and loses life-giving vitality. Likewise, energy can be forced into a straight line, such as by a long hallway, where it can gain momentum and become uncomfortable or destructive. *Chi* is the positive, calm energy in between the two extremes of sha. To keep things in balance, positive energy needs to flow unimpeded through the home.

The art of feng shui is a process of assessing and neutralizing negative energy and fostering positive energy. Balancing the energy in the home lays the foundation for cultivating a comfortable ambience. It also provides us with support for dealing with personal issues.

The Three A's of Working with Energy

Now that we know energy needs to be kept in balance, where do we start? With the three A's: awareness, adjustment, and activation. First, be aware of and assess your surroundings. Take a few minutes to sit quietly in a room. If something doesn't feel right, look for a source of negative energy, then make an adjustment.

In feng shui, an adjustment to counteract negativity is called a *cure*. Feng shui cures with essential oils can be applied in several ways using a reed diffuser, a candle, or an aromatic salt.

It is often helpful to begin your assessment by looking outside your home. The artificial environments of towns and cities with busy roads can have a strong impact on the energy of our homes. Assess how energy flows toward your house or apartment building. If you live on a busy street, you may be bombarded with fast-moving energy that can affect or drain the positive energy from your home. If you live on a cul de sac, energy may be stagnating and creating a pool of negativity. While we usually cannot change the source of negative energy from outside, we can deal with it from inside by placing a cure on a windowsill or somewhere near the wall in the direction of the problem.

· · · · · · · ·

Assess the Energy inside Your Home

After looking outside, assess how energy enters and moves through your home. In feng shui, the front door is regarded as the main entry point for energy. Any blockage here will inhibit positive energy from entering and circulating freely to create a balanced environment. Blessings and abundance could get stuck on your doorstep instead of coming into your life. A cure placed near the front door can help regulate the flow of energy.

Continue through your home. Look for areas where energy can get boxed in or where it may speed up. Place a cure in the area where you want to change and balance the energy.

Energy from the environment isn't the only thing to be aware of. Sometimes we carry tension home with us from work, and sometimes a conflict in the family can create unsettled energy. In addition, a room may just feel "off" without an apparent reason. In these situations, use a calming cure to change the quality of the energy.

The time of year and weather can also affect the energy of our homes. During the excitement of the holiday season, with an increase in family and friends visiting, we may need to tone down the energy to avoid an atmosphere of chaos. However, after the holidays and especially in northern areas where it is cold and dark, we may want to ratchet up the level of energy.

The key to success is to start small. Don't try to take on the whole house at once. Start with any exterior source of negativity. After that, focus on the front door to make sure positive energy is coming in. Follow that by working individually with one room or one area within a room. Take your time, make an adjustment, and then assess the results.

The Aromatic Salt Cure

Salt is important for its purifying properties. In energy work, it neutralizes negativity and clears the way for positive energy to flow. Salt and salt water cures are commonly used in traditional feng shui, but they can be messy. While salt lamps are often used, they can act as dehumidifiers, drying the environment, or in high humidity they can drip salt. However, all is not lost, because we can simply whip up a batch of extra-strong bath salts. Be sure to label the jar as "feng shui salts" so you don't inadvertently use them in the bath.

Use a decorative glass jar with a tight lid so you can store the salts until they are needed. Tie a ribbon around the jar to add color, or add a drop or two of natural food coloring when mixing the salts. Depending on the strength of the essential oil or blend, you may need to adjust the amount. Table 15.1 provides a list of oils that are effective for calming, stimulating, and balancing energy. The carrier oil in the feng shui salts recipe helps to distribute the essential oils.

Feng Shui Salts

1 cup Epsom or sea salts

⅓–½ cup carrier oil

1–1½ teaspoons essential oil or blend

Place the salts in a glass or ceramic bowl. Combine the carrier and essential oils and mix thoroughly. Store in a jar with a tight-fitting lid when the scent is not needed.

Table 15.1 Essential Oils for Aromatic Feng Shui

To Calm Energy
Amyris, caraway seed, cardamom, citronella, clary sage, cypress, elemi, geranium, lavender, mandarin, manuka, neroli, palmarosa, patchouli, sage, sandalwood, vetiver, ylang-ylang
To Balance Energy
Amyris, angelica (seed), cajeput, cardamom, carrot seed, chamomile, clary sage, frankincense, geranium, lavender, lemon balm, marjoram, myrrh, petitgrain, ravintsara, rose, tea tree
To Stimulate Energy
Angelica (root), anise seed, basil, bay laurel, bergamot, black pepper, cedarwood, cinnamon leaf, clove bud, coriander, eucalyptus, fennel, fir needle, ginger, grapefruit, helichrysum, hyssop, juniper berry, lemon, lemongrass, lime, niaouli, orange, patchouli, peppermint, pine, rosemary, spearmint, thyme

To slow down fast-moving energy or remove negativity, place a reed diffuser, a candle, or an open jar of feng shui salts with the appropriate essential oil or blend in that area of your home. When you sense that the energy is better, you can remove it or replace it with a diffuser, candle, or jar of salts containing any of the balancing oils. Do the same with the stimulating oils when you need to get energy moving. You may notice that some essential oils, such as amyris and geranium, can do double duty for both calming and balancing energy.

Using a candle may not always be appropriate for safety reasons, depending on where you need to place it. However, if its scent is strong, you may not need to light it for its aroma to be effective.

For problems originating outside the home, place your salt jar or other cure item in a window or along the wall in the direction of the problem. Occasionally, negative energy may be caused by a neighbor. In this situation, place a jar of salts with balancing oils on a windowsill or on a table near a window that faces your neighbor's house and leave it there.

As mentioned, energy is constantly changing, but by taking a little time to assess what is going on in your home, you can keep positive energy flowing. The next two parts provide an in-depth exploration of essential oils, carrier oils, and other important ingredients.

• • • • • • • •

PART SIX

Essential Oil Profiles

This part of the book provides in-depth profiles of over sixty essential oils. Each profile contains background information on the plant and its historical uses to give you a perspective on how the plants and oils have been important in the past. In some cases, these details can deepen your appreciation of essential oils or spark your imagination for unique ways of using them. Designed to put everything at your fingertips, each profile contains the following information:

- The common, botanical, and other name(s) of the plant
- A description of the oil and its viscosity to aid in measuring drops
- Approximate shelf life to determine how much oil to purchase and how long it may last
- Specific precautions and other pertinent information

Sections within each profile correspond to the previous parts of this book to provide a holistic approach for using the essential oil. These include the following:

- A description of the scent, along with other oils that mix well with it
- Blending details, such as scent group, perfume note, initial strength, and sun signs
- A listing of the ailments and conditions it can be used for and remedy suggestions
- Personal care products and how to personalize them
- Aromatherapy methods for well-being
- How to use the oil to work with the chakras
- Spiritual and magical applications of the oil

• • • • • • • •

- Uses for freshening and cleaning the home and pest control
- Aromatic feng shui ideas to balance or adjust the energy of your home

✋ Amyris ✋

BOTANICAL NAME: *Amyris balsamifera* syn. *Schimmelia oleifera*
ALSO KNOWN AS: Candlewood, torchwood, West Indian sandalwood, white rosewood

Amyris was formerly known as West Indian sandalwood until the late nineteenth century, when it was discovered to have no relation to the East Indian or true sandalwood (*Santalum album*). In the past, amyris was frequently used in perfumery as a substitute for true sandalwood because it was less expensive. Today, the reason to substitute it for sandalwood is ecological because *Santalum album* is under threat. Several other names applied to amyris relate to the practice of using its resinous wood as torches for traveling or fishing at night. It was also common to burn small pieces of the fragrant wood as incense. Today, amyris is most often used as a fixative in perfumery.

Native to the West Indies and South America, amyris is a small bushy tree with pointed oval leaves. Small white flowers grow in clusters and produce blackish-blue berries. The genus name *Amyris* is derived from the Greek *amyon*, meaning "sweet oil" or "unguent." [15]

Oil Description and Precautions
Amyris is a pale yellow oil produced by steam distillation of the wood and branches. It has a thick viscosity and an approximate shelf life of two to three years or slightly longer. There are no known precautions for this oil.

Blending for Scent
The scent of amyris is woody and cedar-like, with warm vanilla undertones. Other oils that blend well with it include cedarwood, citronella, ginger, lavender, palmarosa, rose, and ylang-ylang.

Scent Group	Perfume Note	Initial Strength	Sun Sign
Woody	Base	Mild	Libra

Medicinal Remedies
Amyris is used for anxiety, muscle aches and pains, and stress.

15. *Webster's Third New International Dictionary of the English Language* (1981), s.v. "amyris," 75.

Although this essential oil is most often used in perfumery, it has been found to help alleviate stress and relieve anxiety. To help soothe frazzled nerves and unwind after a stressful day, diffuse 3 parts amyris, 2 parts geranium, and 1 part lemon balm.

The balsamic properties of amyris also make it effective for loosening tight muscles, especially after sports or other physical exertion. Mix 6 drops of amyris, 5 drops of lavender, and 3 drops of ginger in an ounce of carrier oil for an effective massage blend.

Personal Care and Well-Being

This oil is an aid for toning the skin and is especially helpful for mature complexions to regenerate cells and combat wrinkles. Its mildly antiseptic properties aid in soothing the occasional pimple outbreak. Combine amyris with lavender to make a moisturizer that will soften and smooth your skin.

Amyris Complexion Care Moisturizer

1 tablespoon cocoa butter, grated or shaved

1–1 ½ tablespoons coconut oil

8–14 drops essential oil or blend

Boil a little water in a saucepan and remove it from the heat. Place the cocoa butter and coconut oil in a jar, set it in the water, and stir until the butter melts. Set the jar aside and let it cool to room temperature. Repeat the heating process and let the mixture cool to room temperature again. Add the essential oil and mix thoroughly. Place the jar in the refrigerator for five or six hours. Let it warm to room temperature before using or storing.

When used in a diffuser or candle, amyris fosters a peaceful, calming atmosphere. It is also an aid for balancing moods and improving mental clarity. The scent of amyris supports and enhances spiritual practices too.

For energy work, amyris activates the sacral and throat chakras. When used for candle magic, it aids in removing negative energy as well as things you no longer need in your life. Use amyris in a reed diffuser in your bedroom to enhance dream work, or burn an amyris candle during past-life work.

For the Home

When practicing aromatic feng shui, use amyris in areas where you want to slow down fast-moving energy. This oil is also instrumental in keeping the energy of a home balanced.

• • • • • • • •

❧ Angelica ☙

BOTANICAL NAME: *Angelica archangelica*

ALSO KNOWN AS: archangel, angelic herb, European angelica, garden angelica, wild celery

Reaching five to eight feet tall, angelica is best described as statuesque. Its purple stems support large coarsely toothed leaves and umbels (umbrella-shaped clusters) of greenish-white honey-scented flowers. In medieval Latin, this plant was called *herba angelica* (angelic herb) because it was believed to protect against the plague like a guardian angel.

Angelica was a prized medicinal herb for centuries and was used in a range of remedies during the Middle Ages and Renaissance. In the tropics, the essential oil of angelica was mixed with quinine for a potent treatment of malaria. By the late seventeenth century, angelica's wide use as a medicinal herb declined, although it was still common in home remedies in England well into the early twentieth century. Today, it has made a comeback with the popularity of herbal remedies.

Oil Description and Precautions

Steam distillation is used to obtain two oils from angelica. The oil from the root is colorless or pale yellow and turns yellowish brown as it ages. Oil from the seeds is colorless. Both oils have a thin viscosity and an approximate shelf life between nine and twelve months.

Avoid using both angelica oils during pregnancy; diabetics should avoid them too. Essential oil from the root is phototoxic. An oil called *white angelica* should not be confused with the essential oils from the angelica plant. White angelica is a blend of oils that, surprisingly, does not contain angelica.

Blending for Scent

Angelica root oil has a rich herbaceous, earthy scent. Other oils that blend well with it include bergamot, clary sage, lemon, lemon balm, lime, orange, patchouli, and vetiver. The seed oil is also herbaceous and earthy but has a hint of spice. Oils that blend well with it include bay laurel, ginger, lavender, and pine.

	Scent Group	Perfume Note	Initial Strength	Sun Signs
Root oil	Herbaceous	Middle to base	Strong	Aries, Leo
Seed oil		Middle to top	Medium	

Medicinal Remedies

Both types of angelica oil are used for anxiety, arthritis, bronchitis, colds, coughs, gout, headaches, indigestion, migraines, psoriasis, and stress.

• • • • • • • •

Because the oil made from the root has a stronger scent and is often more readily available than the seed oil, it tends to be used more often in recipes. However, both oils are effective and worth exploring.

To relieve anxiety, nervous tension, headache, or stress, use angelica on its own in a diffuser or mix it in equal amounts with lavender and lemon balm. Used as a steam inhalation, angelica helps relieve colds, flu, and associated respiratory ailments. To give angelica a boost, combine it with cypress or manuka.

On its own or with other essential oils, angelica eases the pain and joint stiffness of arthritis. The following massage blend can be used to make bath salts for a soothing soak in the tub, too.

Warming Relief Angelica Massage Oil

2 tablespoons carrier oil

5 drops angelica essential oil

4 drops rosemary essential oil

3 drops lemon essential oil

Combine all the oils and swirl gently to mix. Store leftover oil in a bottle with a tight-fitting cap.

Angelica is effective for treating psoriasis. Mix 1 drop each of angelica and bergamot with a teaspoon of coconut or evening primrose carrier oil. Gently dab the mixture on the affected areas.

Working as an expectorant, angelica helps to ease respiratory problems, especially chronic bronchitis. For an effective steam inhalation, combine 3 drops of angelica, 2 drops of lemon, and 1 drop of pine.

Personal Care and Well-Being

Angelica stimulates the skin and helps brighten a dull complexion. Use the seed oil to make a skin toner. Angelica's soothing qualities make it suitable for sensitive skin. If you use the root oil, wait at least twelve hours before going out in the sun, as it is phototoxic and can irritate the skin like a sunburn.

Creating a peaceful atmosphere, angelica helps to balance moods, cope with life's challenges, and ease sorrow. Diffuse 2 parts each of angelica and mandarin and 1 part sandalwood for a revitalizing scent to ease mental fatigue and nervous tension.

Use angelica root oil to activate the root chakra, and the seed oil for the third eye and crown chakras. Either type of angelica oil is effective to ground and center energy for meditation and prayer. Angelica also provides spiritual support. Use it to consecrate your altar or sacred space and to aid you in sending healing prayers. As its name suggests, it is helpful for connecting with angelic energy. In candle magic, use the root or seed oil to attract success for important endeavors or to banish what you no longer need in your life. Angelica also supports dream work.

• • • • • • • •

For the Home

Just as angelica seeds can be burned as incense, the essential oil used in a diffuser freshens and deodorizes the air. For feng shui, use angelica root oil in an area where you need to stimulate energy and get it moving. Afterward, use the seed oil for balance.

❧ Anise Seed ❧

Botanical name: *Pimpinella anisum* syn. *Anisum officinalis*

Also known as: aniseed, sweet cumin

Anise is an herb that looks like a small spindly version of Queen Anne's lace. It has feathery leaves and umbels of delicate white or yellowish flowers. Valued since ancient times, anise seed has been cultivated in Egypt for approximately four thousand years.[16] Its common name comes from the Latin *anisun*, which was derived from the Arab name for the plant, *anysum*.[17] The ancient Greeks and Romans used anise in after-dinner cakes to aid digestion. Greek philosopher Theophrastus (c. 372–c. 288 BCE) noted that keeping anise seeds by one's bed at night resulted in sweet dreams.

As in the past, anise is used to flavor a wide variety of liqueurs, including Benedictine, Chartreuse, ouzo, and, of course, anisette. It should not be confused with star anise essential oil, which is produced from the fruit of the Chinese star anise tree (*Illicium verum*).

Oil Description and Precautions

Steam distillation of anise seeds produces a pale yellow oil with a thin viscosity. It has an approximate shelf life of two to three years. Avoid anise seed oil during pregnancy and while breastfeeding; avoid with cancer or liver disease; may cause skin irritation or dermatitis; avoid use on allergic or inflamed skin; do not use on children under six years old; use in moderation.

Blending for Scent

Anise seed has a spicy, sweet, and licorice-like scent. Some of the oils that blend well with it include caraway seed, cardamom, coriander, mandarin, petitgrain, and rose.

Scent Group	Perfume Note	Initial Strength	Sun Signs
Spicy	Top	Strong	Aquarius, Pisces, Gemini, Leo, Sagittarius

16. Chevallier, *The Encyclopedia of Medicinal Plants*, 247.

17. Cumo, ed., *Encyclopedia of Cultivated Plants*, 27.

Medicinal Remedies

Anise seed essential oil is used for anxiety, arthritis, bronchitis, colds, coughs, flu, hangover, indigestion, menopausal discomforts, menstrual cramps, muscle aches and pains, nausea, stress, vertigo, and whooping cough.

Anise seed is a decongestant that brings comforting relief for respiratory issues related to colds, flu, and coughs. Place a couple of drops in a teaspoon of carrier oil to make a quick and easy chest rub. Anise seed's expectorant properties make it effective for bronchitis and whooping cough. When used for a steam inhalation, it opens the nasal and bronchial airways. Simply place 6 or 7 drops in a quart of steaming water. In the bath or shower, anise seed provides warming relief from cold and flu symptoms.

Anise Seed Shower Melts

½ cup cocoa butter, grated or shaved

4 tablespoons sunflower carrier oil

20 drops anise seed essential oil

20 drops lemon essential oil

12 drops pine essential oil

Bring a saucepan of water to a boil and remove from the heat. Place the cocoa butter and sunflower oil in a jar in the water. Stir until the butter melts. Let the mixture cool to room temperature, then add the essential oils. Pour the mixture into mini cupcake liners or candy molds. Place in the refrigerator for five or six hours, then remove. To use, place one melt on the floor of the shower.

To reduce stress and promote restful sleep, mix anise seed in equal parts with lavender and lemon balm to diffuse in the bedroom before bedtime. Alternatively, sprinkle a few drops of these oils on the bedsheets.

Personal Care and Well-Being

Soothing and comforting, anise seed helps us to balance our emotions and cope with changes. Its uplifting scent fosters a general sense of well-being. Use anise seed when working with the sacral, heart, or third eye chakras. Spiritually, this oil can be used to consecrate an altar or sacred space. It also supports meditation. When working with candle magic, use anise seed to remove negative energy, to attract love or luck, and to foster happiness. Anise seed is also instrumental in dream work.

· · · · · · ·

For the Home

The antibacterial properties of anise seed make it an ideal choice for an air freshener and room deodorizer. Combine it with orange or pine for a clean, refreshing scent that does more than make a room smell nice. For aromatic feng shui, use anise seed to stimulate energy, especially in an area of the house where the flow may be impeded or blocked.

✺ Basil ✺

BOTANICAL NAME: *Ocimum basilicum*

ALSO KNOWN AS: Common basil, French basil, Genovese basil, sweet basil

Basil is a bushy plant that reaches one to two feet tall. Its oval leaves have a distinctive downward curl and prominent veins. The leaves are yellow green to dark green and very fragrant. White, pink, or purple flowers grow at the tops of stems. Basil's genus and species names were derived from the Greek words for "smell" and "royal," respectively.[18] The French called it *herbe royale*. Basil is thought to have come from the Indian plant holy basil (*Ocimum sanctum*) and transported to Greece by Alexander the Great.

The ancient Egyptians, Greeks, and Romans used basil for medicinal and culinary purposes. Greek physician Pedanius Dioscorides (c. 40–90 CE) made note of it in his writing. By the early sixteenth century, basil was being grown in northern Europe and England. During the Middle Ages, it was used as a strewing herb, scattered on floors to help freshen and clear the air and for pest control. By the late sixteenth century, the Spanish had transported basil to North America.

Oil Description and Precautions

Basil leaves and flower tops are steam-distilled, producing a thin, colorless to pale yellow oil. It has an approximate shelf life of two to three years. Avoid this oil during pregnancy; use in moderation and avoid prolonged use; may cause dermal irritation.

Blending for Scent

Initially anise-like, basil's pungent scent is herbaceous and sweetly spicy. Some of the oils that blend well with it include black pepper, citronella, lemon, lemongrass, marjoram, peppermint, and spearmint.

Scent Group	Perfume Note	Initial Strength	Sun Signs
Herbaceous	Middle to top	Strong to very strong	Aries, Leo, Scorpio

18. Heilmeyer, *Ancient Herbs*, 128.

• • • • • • • •

Medicinal Remedies

This essential oil is used for anxiety, arthritis, bronchitis, circulation, colds, coughs, depression, earaches, fainting, fever, flu, gout, headaches, insect bites and stings, insomnia, migraines, muscle aches and pains, nausea, sinus infection, and stress.

Basil relieves muscle aches and pains and is especially effective after overexertion. It works well on its own, or it can be combined with lavender and marjoram for an aromatic treat that is equally soothing for the mind. Combining basil with marjoram and rosemary also works well for sore muscles.

Basil Muscle-Soothing Oil

2 tablespoons St. John's wort carrier oil

5 drops basil essential oil

5 drops lavender essential oil

3 drops marjoram essential oil

Combine all the oils and swirl to mix. Store any leftover oil in a bottle with a tight-fitting cap.

Basil's antibacterial and antiviral properties make it effective in treating respiratory ailments, including sinus infections. Diffuse 2 parts basil with 1 part each of pine and spearmint, or use these oils for a steam inhalation. To relieve insect bites, put 2 or 3 drops of basil in a teaspoon of carrier oil and apply to the area. Basil is especially effective for mosquito bites and wasp stings.

To ease anxiety, place 4 drops of basil and 3 drops each of clary sage and chamomile (Roman) in an inhaler to use as needed. A few drops of basil on a tissue helps to revive someone who has fainted.

Personal Care and Well-Being

Along with rosemary, basil can be used for a scalp treatment to help stimulate hair growth. Use 1 drop each in a teaspoon of carrier oil to massage into the scalp at bedtime. Leave it on overnight, then shampoo in the morning. Continue using the preparation until new growth begins.

Basil helps us to balance the emotions and cope with changes. Diffuse it in equal amounts with bergamot and lavender to lift your mood. Basil also helps when dealing with grief after the death of a loved one. When you need to concentrate and study, place a couple of drops in the melted wax of a pillar candle to help clear your head and focus your mind. This oil also fosters a sense of peace. Combine it in equal amounts with lemon and juniper berry to help relieve fatigue and nervous tension. Basil activates the energy of the solar plexus and throat chakras.

For spiritual purposes, basil aids in sending healing prayers and connecting with angels. Because it may have come from the holy basil plant, it is instrumental for cleaning and consecrating an altar.

. . . .

When used in candle magic, basil removes negativity and helps attract prosperity and success. Also use it to foster love or invite happiness into your life.

For the Home

Effective for treating mosquito bites and wasp stings, basil also helps to repel these pests. Use it in a reed diffuser near a window or in candles for outdoor gatherings. For aromatic feng shui, basil is effective for stimulating and moving energy.

✎ Bay Laurel ✎

BOTANICAL NAME: *Laurus nobilis*

ALSO KNOWN AS: Bay tree, Roman laurel, sweet bay, true bay

In addition to the use of bay leaves in soups and stews, this plant may be familiar as a small potted tree that is often cut into pom-poms or other topiary shapes. Its leathery dark green leaves are oval and sharply pointed. Small oval berries turn blue-black when ripe.

Bay's botanical name comes from the Latin *laurus*, meaning "to praise" or "to honor," and *nobilis*, "renowned." [19] It was customary for ancient Greeks and Romans to honor people of accomplishment with crowns of bay laurel. In addition to decorating shrines and other public spaces with bay, the leaves were used for culinary and medicinal purposes and as an insect repellent. Abbess Hildegard of Bingen (1098–1179) and herbalist Nicholas Culpeper highly recommended bay laurel for a range of ailments.

Oil Description and Precautions

The leaves and small branches are steam-distilled, producing a greenish-yellow oil. It has a thin viscosity and an approximate shelf life of two to three years. Do not use bay laurel when taking painkillers or sedative medications; avoid during pregnancy and when nursing; may cause sensitization or dermal irritation in some; use in moderation. As mentioned in chapter 4, West Indian bay (*Pimenta racemosa*) is often simply called *bay* and should not be confused with bay laurel, as it has different uses and precautions.

Blending for Scent

Bay laurel has a fresh herbaceous and slightly camphoraceous scent. Some of the oils that blend well with it include bergamot, clary sage, eucalyptus (blue), frankincense, ginger, juniper berry, lavender, lemon, and rosemary.

Scent Group	Perfume Note	Initial Strength	Sun Signs
Herbaceous	Middle to top	Medium	Gemini, Leo, Pisces

19. Harrison, *Latin for Gardeners*, 120.

Medicinal Remedies

Bay laurel is used for arthritis, athlete's foot, bruises, colds, eczema, fever, flu, indigestion, jock itch, psoriasis, rashes, sore throat, sprains and strains, and tonsillitis.

With antiviral and antibacterial properties, bay laurel is helpful for relieving cold and flu symptoms. Use it in a steam inhalation to soothe inflammation, ease nasal congestion, and help clear respiratory airways. Combine bay laurel with rosemary to make a warming chest rub.

Soothing Bay and Rosemary Chest Rub

¼ ounce beeswax

3½ tablespoons carrier oil or blend

17 drops bay laurel essential oil

10 drops rosemary essential oil

Place the beeswax and carrier oil in a jar in a saucepan of water. Warm it over low heat, stirring until the wax melts. Remove it from the heat and let the mixture cool to room temperature before adding the essential oils. Test the thickness of the mixture and adjust if necessary. Let it cool completely before using or storing.

Bay laurel works well in a steam inhalation to relieve cold and flu symptoms. Add 5 to 6 drops to a quart of boiling water. This oil can also be used in a nasal inhaler that you can take with you for relief wherever you go. For an extra-powerful inhaler blend, use 5 drops each of bay laurel and fir needle and 2 drops of ginger.

The analgesic properties of bay laurel help relieve the stiffness and pain of arthritis. Combine 3 drops of bay with 2 drops each of eucalyptus (blue) and juniper berry in a tablespoon of carrier oil for a warming massage. Combine it with chamomile and helichrysum to soothe sprains and reduce bruising.

Personal Care and Well-Being

Bay laurel helps keep hair healthy and is especially good for both dry and oily hair. For dandruff control, mix 3 to 4 drops in a tablespoon of carrier oil and massage into the scalp. Leave it on for about fifteen minutes, then shampoo and rinse well. It also aids hair growth.

The uplifting scent of bay laurel is an aid for emotional balance. Diffuse it or put a few drops in the melted wax of a pillar candle to clear the head and aid concentration. Bay also fosters peace of mind. For energy work, it stimulates the solar plexus and third eye chakras. Bay laurel supports spiritual practices and helps in sending healing prayers. It is also ideal for consecrating an altar. In candle magic, bay aids in attracting abundance and prosperity. It is also helpful for achieving success, especially when seeking justice. Sprinkle a few drops of bay laurel on your pillow before bed to support dream work.

· · · · · · · ·

For the Home

Bay laurel is useful as an insect repellent and is especially effective against moths. Liberally sprinkle equal amounts of bay laurel, eucalyptus (blue), and lavender on a few cotton balls, then place them in the closet or area where moths have been a problem. With its antibacterial and antifungal properties, bay laurel works well in a diffuser to clean and freshen the air. For aromatic feng shui, use it wherever you need to get energy moving.

✺ Bergamot ✺

BOTANICAL NAME: *Citrus bergamia* syn. *C. aurantium* var. *bergamia*

ALSO KNOWN AS: Bergamot orange

Bergamot is believed to be a hybrid of the lemon (*C. limon*) and bitter orange (*C. aurantium*). Cultivated in the Mediterranean region since the seventeenth century, it was first used as an ornamental garden plant. It has fragrant white flowers that grow in clusters and smooth oval leaves. Its yellow, slightly pear-shaped fruit has been called *bergamotta oranges* and *bergamotta pears*.

Although its name is often said to have come from the town of Bergamo in northern Italy, the tree was known as bergamotta long before it was grown in that area. Other contenders for the name are Berga, where it was grown near Barcelona, Spain, and the Turkish word *beg-armudi*, which means "pear of the prince."[20] The essential oil of this fruit has been popular in perfumery since the eighteenth century. One of the plant's culinary uses is to give Earl Grey tea its distinctive flavor.

Oil Description and Precautions

Cold-pressing the fruit peel produces a greenish-yellow oil with a thin viscosity. Unlike other citrus oils, bergamot has an approximate shelf life of two to three years. Bergamot is phototoxic. This oil should not be confused with the essential oil from the herb bergamot mint (*Mentha citrata*).

Blending for Scent

Bergamot has a citrusy sweet and slightly floral scent. Some of the oils that blend well with it include basil, chamomile (German), coriander, cypress, geranium, ginger, juniper berry, rose, sandalwood, and vetiver.

Scent Group	Perfume Note	Initial Strength	Sun Signs
Citrus	Top	Mild	Gemini, Virgo

20. Dugo and Bonaccorsi, eds., *Citrus Bergamia*, 3.

· · · · · · · ·

Medicinal Remedies

Bergamot is used for acne, anxiety, blisters, boils, chicken pox, cold sores, colds, cuts and scrapes, depression, eczema, fever, flu, insect bites and stings, jet lag, laryngitis, premenstrual syndrome (PMS), psoriasis, rashes, scabies, seasonal affective disorder (SAD), sore throat, stress, tonsillitis, and varicose veins.

With analgesic and antibacterial properties, bergamot is effective for fighting infection and treating a range of ailments. Combine 2 drops of bergamot with 1 drop of lemon in a teaspoon of carrier oil to dab on blisters, cold sores, and other skin eruptions. To make a compress for heat rash, use 3 drops each of the same oils in a tablespoon of carrier oil, then add it to a quart of cool water. To soothe and heal insect bites and stings, combine bergamot with manuka.

Bergamot is also effective in treating colds, flu, and throat problems. Mix 3 drops each of bergamot and spearmint and 1 drop of thyme in a quart of water for a steam inhalation. This combination of essential oils is also good to diffuse in a sickroom to clear the air.

Personal Care and Well-Being

Bergamot is cleansing and soothing for the skin. Its antiseptic properties make it particularly effective as an astringent for oily skin, acne, and pimple outbreaks. For an all-over clean, use it to make a body scrub. Bergamot also works well in deodorant and body powder to fight odor.

The uplifting scent of bergamot is especially popular in aromatherapy for balancing the emotions, calming tension, and dealing with depression. Combine 6 drops of bergamot and 2 drops each of lavender and cypress in a tealight diffuser or add them to the melted wax of a pillar candle. Diffuse bergamot on its own for support when dealing with grief. The refreshing scent of bergamot also helps to calm anger.

Bergamot is especially calming when combined with clary sage and lavender. For a mood lift during PMS, combine it with clary and geranium. Diffuse bergamot before bedtime to aid in getting a restful night's sleep. This oil fosters a sense of well-being and peace. Combine it with a little peppermint when you need to concentrate.

For energy work, use bergamot to activate and balance the sacral, heart, and throat chakras. It also provides support for meditation and spiritual practices. In candle magic, use bergamot to attract love or luck, reach goals, or help when you are seeking justice. It also supports dream work.

For the Home

For aromatic feng shui, use bergamot to get energy moving wherever it feels sluggish or bogged down. Like other citrus oils, bergamot not only smells fresh and clean but also makes a good household cleaner, especially for glass.

Bergamot Glass Cleaner

1½ cup white vinegar

½ cup water

8 drops bergamot essential oil

5 drops orange essential oil

5 drops lemon essential oil

Combine all ingredients in a spray bottle and shake well. Use the mixture on windows and mirrors as you would any other glass cleaner.

✺ Black Pepper ✺

BOTANICAL NAME: *Piper nigrum*

Indigenous to southwestern India, this woody climbing vine can grow up to sixteen feet long. It has small white flowers and dark green heart-shaped leaves. Its red berries turn black as they ripen, becoming the familiar peppercorn when dried. Although we may consider pepper as extremely common, in the past it was regarded as the king of spices. Black pepper was used medicinally in China, India, and Egypt for thousands of years. Although it was highly prized by the ancient Greeks and Romans for culinary purposes, their physicians wrote about pepper's use in remedies. It was also said to be an aphrodisiac.

An important trade commodity, pepper became the must-have food flavoring throughout Europe. This put English and Dutch traders in a race to find a water route to the Far East so they could cut out the middlemen in the overland routes. In 1180, specialized merchants called *pepperers* formed a guild in London.[21] During the Middle Ages, pepper was so valuable that it served as payment for dowries and taxes.

Oil Description and Precautions

The dried unripe fruit is steam-distilled, producing a clear to slightly yellowish-green oil. It has a thin viscosity and a shelf life of two to three years or slightly longer. This essential oil may cause skin irritation; avoid during pregnancy and while breastfeeding; not compatible with homeopathic treatment; use in moderation; use in low dilution; do not use on children under six years old.

Blending for Scent

Black pepper has a pungently spicy and slightly woody scent. Unlike ground pepper, the essential oil does not cause sneezing. Some of the oils that blend well with it include clary sage, clove bud, coriander, fennel, frankincense, grapefruit, lavender, lemon, lime, and ylang-ylang.

21. Weiss, *Spice Crops*, 156.

Scent Group	Perfume Note	Initial Strength	Sun Sign
Spicy	Middle to base	Strong	Aries

Medicinal Remedies

This essential oil is used for anxiety, arthritis, chilblains, circulation, colds, constipation, fainting, fever, flu, indigestion, muscle aches and pains, nausea, sprains and strains, stress, and tendonitis.

The analgesic properties of black pepper make it ideal for sore muscles and arthritic joint pain. Combine 2 drops each of black pepper, coriander, and juniper berry in an ounce of carrier oil for a soothing massage. As an anti-inflammatory, black pepper also aids in healing sprains and strains. Because it stimulates circulation, massaging with black pepper can warm up cold feet and hands.

Black Pepper Foot Warming Blend

1 teaspoon carrier oil

1 drop black pepper essential oil

Mix oils thoroughly before applying. Store any leftover oil in a bottle with a tight-fitting lid.

For a warming footbath, combine 3 drops of black pepper with a tablespoon of carrier oil and add it to a basin of comfortably warm water. The antimicrobial and antiseptic properties of this oil are an aid for colds and flu. Use 2 drops of black pepper and 1 drop each of neroli and pine in a quart of water for a steam inhalation to alleviate the symptoms. To deal with anxiety and stress, diffuse 2 parts palmarosa and 1 part each of black pepper and ylang-ylang.

Personal Care and Well-Being

Just as black pepper aids in the relief of anxiety and stress, it also helps with emotional issues such as dealing with changes and ratcheting down anger. Diffuse 1 part black pepper and 2 parts each of lemon and cedarwood for emotional support. Black pepper also stimulates and clears the mind and supports concentration. Because this oil often causes irritation, it is not used in skin or hair care.

For energy work, use black pepper to activate the solar plexus and third eye chakras. This oil's grounding and centering properties make it helpful when preparing for meditation or prayer. Spiritually, it is also effective for consecrating an altar or shrine and sending healing prayers. When working with candle magic, this oil helps to remove negative energy, find justice, and achieve success. Pepper is also helpful for dream work.

· · · · · · · ·

For the Home

In the home, black pepper essential oil is effective for stimulating energy. Use it in feng shui salts wherever the energy feels stagnant or blocked.

❧ Cajeput ❧

BOTANICAL NAME: *Melaleuca leucadendron* syn. *M. cajuputi, M. minor*
ALSO KNOWN AS: Paperbark tree, swamp tea tree, white tea tree, white wood

Reaching a height of over a hundred feet, this tree's distinctive feature is its whitish bark that peels in paperlike flakes. Its evergreen leaves are thick and pointed. Clusters of white flowers grow in spikes that resemble bottlebrushes. Native to Southeast Asia, cajeput was highly valued for its medicinal uses. During the seventeenth century, Dutch trading companies introduced it into Europe, where it became part of the pharmacist's arsenal for many centuries. Today it is cultivated for its essential oil and timber. Cajeput is a close cousin of tea tree (*M. alternifolia*).

From Latin, its species name, *leucadendron*, means "white tree."[22] Its common name is most likely a corruption of the Indonesian name for the tree, *kayu putih*, which also means "white tree."[23]

Oil Description and Precautions

Steam distillation of the leaves and twigs produces a pale yellow-green oil with a thin viscosity. It has an approximate shelf life of twelve to eighteen months. Cajeput may cause skin irritation; do not use on children under six years old.

Blending for Scent

Cajeput has a camphoraceous and slightly fruity, sweet scent. Some oils that blend well with it include bergamot, clove bud, geranium, lavender, rosemary, and thyme.

Scent Group	Perfume Note	Initial Strength	Sun Sign
Woody	Middle to top	Medium to strong	Sagittarius

Medicinal Remedies

Cajeput essential oil is used for acne, arthritis, asthma, athlete's foot, bronchitis, bursitis, circulation, colds, coughs, earaches, eczema, flu, head lice, headaches, insect bites and stings, laryngitis, muscle aches and pains, scabies, sinus infection, sore throat, vaginal infections, and warts.

Like its cousin tea tree, cajeput is an aid in fighting certain fungal infections. For warts, combine 2 drops of cajeput and 3 drops each of lemon and cedarwood (Virginia) in a tablespoon

---

22. Harrison, *Latin for Gardeners*, 123.
23. Southwell and Lowe, eds., *Tea Tree*, 213.

of carrier oil. Apply 1 or 2 drops of the blend to the wart three times a day and keep it covered with an adhesive bandage. For athlete's foot, cajeput can be used on its own with 2 drops in a teaspoon of carrier oil, or it can be combined with other essential oils to make a salve.

Cajeput Athlete's Foot Salve

3 tablespoons cocoa butter, grated or shaved

2 tablespoons carrier oil or blend

18 drops cajeput essential oil

15 drops eucalyptus (lemon) essential oil

8 drops bay laurel essential oil

Boil a little water in a saucepan and remove it from the heat. Place the butter and carrier oil in a jar in the water. Stir until the butter melts. Allow the mixture to cool to room temperature. Repeat the heating process, let it cool again, then add the essential oils. Place the jar in the refrigerator for five or six hours. Let the mixture come to room temperature before using or storing.

Cajeput works well as a decongestant to ease respiratory ailments. For a steam inhalation to alleviate symptoms and aid in healing, use 4 drops of cajeput, 3 drops of pine, and 2 drops of lemongrass in a quart of water. This combination of essential oils also works well for a steamy soak in the tub, which will also help open the sinuses. The antiseptic properties of cajeput help to heal a sore throat and soothe laryngitis. Combine cajeput with equal amounts of bergamot and pine in a diffuser to clean the air and breathe easier.

The warming analgesic properties of cajeput are ideal to massage away sore muscles and general stiffness. Combine 5 drops of cajeput, 4 drops of rosemary, and 3 drops of marjoram in an ounce of carrier oil. For a muscle-warming compress, combine 2 drops of cajeput, 3 drops of chamomile (German), and 1 drop of ginger in a quart of comfortably warm water.

Personal Care and Well-Being

The antiseptic properties of cajeput work well in an astringent for oily skin, especially during a pimple outbreak. For combination skin, use cajeput and lavender to make a toner.

This essential oil is an aid for emotional support to keep moods in check and help make a smooth transition during major life changes. To stimulate the mind when concentration is important, diffuse 1 part each of cajeput and eucalyptus (blue) and 2 parts of lemon. This combination of oils will also alleviate mental fatigue.

Cajeput is instrumental in activating the sacral, throat, and third eye chakras. It aids in grounding and centering for meditation and prayer and in sending healing prayers. When engaging in candle magic, cajeput bolsters determination to achieve success.

• • • • • • •

For the Home

For outdoor dining, make candles using a combination of cajeput, lemongrass, and lavender to set the mood and ward off insects. For help indoors, use the same oils in a reed diffuser by an open window. After calming or stimulating the energy flow in your home, use a cajeput candle or feng shui salts to maintain balance.

❧ Caraway Seed ❧

BOTANICAL NAME: *Carum carvi*

ALSO KNOWN AS: Carum, common caraway, Roman cumin

According to archeological evidence, caraway was important to commerce, and its use dates back more than five thousand years.[24] Its genus name comes from the Greek word *karon*, meaning "annual or biennial herb." [25] *Carvi*, the Latin name for caraway, was noted by Roman naturalist Pliny as having come from the Caria region of Asia Minor.[26]

The Greeks and Romans were particularly fond of caraway seeds and used them for medicinal and culinary purposes. In later centuries, caraway essential oil became a valuable commodity in Central Europe, especially Romania, which had a reputation for producing exceptional medicinal herbs. While caraway seeds were valued throughout Europe during the Middle Ages for medicinal purposes, in Northern European countries they became more popular for baking. From Tudor to Victorian times in England, caraway was the most important seed in seed cake, which was a popular teatime treat.

Looking like a small version of Queen Anne's lace, caraway has light green feathery leaves. Its tiny white flowers grow in umbel clusters and bloom during the late summer. Caraway is closely related to anise, dill, and fennel.

Oil Description and Precautions

Steam distillation of the seeds produces a colorless or pale yellow to yellowish-brown oil. It has a thin viscosity and an approximate shelf life of two to three years. Caraway seed essential oil may cause skin irritation in some.

Blending for Scent

This essential oil has a warm, sweet, and spicy scent. Oils that blend well with it include basil, chamomile, coriander, frankincense, ginger, lavender, and orange.

---

24. Kowalchik and Hylton, eds., *Rodale's Illustrated Encyclopedia of Herbs*, 63.
25. Coombes, *Dictionary of Plant Names*, 48.
26. Heilmeyer, *Ancient Herbs*, 30.

Scent Group	Perfume Note	Initial Strength	Sun Sign
Spicy	Middle	Medium to strong	Gemini

Medicinal Remedies

This essential oil is used for asthma, boils, bronchitis, colds, coughs, cuts and scrapes, indigestion, laryngitis, premenstrual syndrome (PMS), and sore throat.

Caraway seed is particularly helpful in a steam inhalation during cold season for easing bronchitis, coughs, and laryngitis. Swish 6 or 7 drops of it into a quart of steaming water. As an alternative, blend 3 drops each of caraway and basil. For relief on the go, use caraway seed in a nasal inhaler.

The antibacterial and antiseptic properties of this oil make it a good choice in a topical ointment for skin problems such as boils, cuts, and scrapes. Combine it with lavender for a boost in effectiveness and a wonderful fragrance.

Fragrant Healing Caraway Seed Ointment

¼ ounce beeswax

3½–4 tablespoons carrier oil or blend

15 drops caraway seed essential oil

12 drops lavender essential oil

Place the beeswax and carrier oil in a jar in a saucepan of water. Warm it over low heat, stirring until the wax melts. Allow the mixture to cool to room temperature before adding the essential oils. Adjust the thickness if necessary. Let it cool completely before using or storing.

Personal Care and Well-Being

Caraway seed works well for oily hair and skin. Make an astringent with 2 ounces of chamomile tea, ½ ounce witch hazel, 5 drops of caraway, 4 drops of chamomile (Roman), and 2 drops of lemon. Dab it on the face with a cotton ball. As a facial steam, caraway stimulates the skin and improves the complexion. For the hair, combine 6 drops of caraway seed with an ounce of apricot kernel carrier oil. Massage it into the scalp and work it through the hair. Leave the mixture on for about ten minutes, then shampoo and rinse well.

For aromatherapy, caraway seed is especially good for calming the nerves and balancing moods. In addition to coping with changes, this oil stimulates the mind and eases mental fatigue. To cultivate a general sense of well-being, combine 5 drops of caraway seed, 4 drops of palmarosa, and 3 drops of basil in a tealight vaporizer.

When working with the chakras, caraway seed activates the sacral, heart, and throat energy centers. Diffuse it for general support during meditation and spiritual practices. In candle magic, caraway seed attracts good luck. It also supports dream work.

For the Home

For aromatic feng shui, use caraway seed in a diffuser or make a jar of salts. Place it wherever you need to mediate and calm the energy flow.

✍ Cardamom ✍

BOTANICAL NAME: *Elettaria cardamomum*

ALSO KNOWN AS: Cardamomi, Indian spice plant

Hailed as the queen of spices, cardamom has been used medicinally since ancient times in China and India. It is still an important ingredient in Traditional Chinese and Ayurvedic medicine. While the ancient Egyptians valued cardamom for perfumes and incense, the Greeks and Romans favored it for culinary and medicinal purposes. A longtime popular culinary spice in India, the Middle East, and Latin America, cardamom has become a trendy spice that is making its way into other cuisines. It is most widely known as an ingredient in chai tea.

Native to India and Sri Lanka, cardamom is a perennial reed-like herb that can grow up to thirteen feet tall. It has long lance-like leaves and yellowish flowers marked with a striking mauve veining pattern. The gray seedpods contain oblong reddish-brown seeds. Its genus name comes from *elettari*, the name of the plant in India. It is called *cardamomum* in Greece.[27]

Oil Description and Precautions

A colorless to pale yellow oil is produced by steam distillation of cardamom seeds. It has a thin viscosity and an approximate shelf life of two to three years. Avoid using this essential oil on children under six years old.

Blending for Scent

Cardamom has a warm, sweetly spicy scent with a woody undertone. Some of the oils that blend well with it include bergamot, caraway seed, cedarwood, cinnamon leaf, clove bud, mandarin, and orange.

Scent Group	Perfume Note	Initial Strength	Sun Signs
Spicy	Middle	Medium to strong	Aries, Cancer, Pisces, Taurus

27. Coombes, *Dictionary of Plant Names*, 78.

Medicinal Remedies

Cardamom essential oil is used for anxiety, constipation, hangover, headaches, indigestion, nausea, premenstrual syndrome (PMS), and stress.

The power of cardamom's healing is mostly centered on the abdomen and stomach. Mix 6 or 7 drops in a tablespoon of carrier oil and gently massage the stomach to help relieve indigestion. Massaging the abdomen in a clockwise (up on the right, down on the left) direction can ease constipation.

Cardamom also alleviates nausea. Place 5 drops of cardamom and 3 drops of peppermint or orange in an inhaler. To combat stress, combine 2 drops each of cardamom and mandarin and 1 drop of cedarwood (Atlas) in a tealight vaporizer. On its own, cardamom is effective for easing morning sickness.

Personal Care and Well-Being

Helping to keep the scalp healthy, cardamom is effective when dealing with dandruff. Add 6 to 8 drops to an ounce of carrier oil, or use 4 drops of cardamom and 3 drops of lemon. Massage it into the scalp, then leave it on for about fifteen minutes. Shampoo and rinse well.

With antibacterial properties, cardamom works well in a deodorant because it kills the bacteria that causes odor. The type of deodorant in the following recipe is applied with the fingertips. You may need to experiment with the quantities to get a consistency you like.

Cardamom Deodorant

¼ cup cornstarch

¼ cup baking soda

¼ cup carrier oil or blend

½ ounce beeswax

20 drops bergamot essential oil

12 drops cardamom essential oil

8 drops ginger essential oil

Combine the dry ingredients and set aside. Place the carrier oil and beeswax in a jar in a saucepan of water and warm over low heat. Stir until the beeswax melts. Let the mixture cool to room temperature before stirring in the essential oils. Use a fork when adding the dry ingredients and mix thoroughly. Store in a jar with a tight-fitting lid.

Uplifting and invigorating, the scent of cardamom helps subdue anger and stabilize mood swings. When you need to focus your attention, diffuse 2 parts cardamom and 1 part each

• • • • • • •

of basil and lemon to clear your mind. Cardamom also aids with mental fatigue and nervous tension.

For energy work, cardamom activates the sacral, solar plexus, and heart chakras. This essential oil is helpful for grounding and centering energy for meditation and in sending healing prayers. For candle magic, cardamom can be used to attract love or banish negative energy.

For the Home

To preserve and polish furniture, combine 2 tablespoons of coconut oil with 5 drops each of cardamom and lemon essential oils. Use a soft cloth to apply, then buff. To help repel insects, use cardamom in a diffuser or add a few drops to the melted wax in a pillar candle. For aromatic feng shui, use cardamom wherever you need to calm energy and maintain balance.

✤ Carrot Seed ✤

BOTANICAL NAME: *Daucus carota*

ALSO KNOWN AS: Bird's nest weed, Queen Anne's lace, wild carrot

Introduced into North America from Europe, Queen Anne's lace is a familiar sight in fields, ditches, and open areas. Growing one to four feet tall, it has feathery leaves and large flower heads that consist of numerous tiny white flowers. Each flower head has a dark reddish-purple floret at the center. According to legend, the center flower represents a drop of Queen Anne's (1665–1714) blood, because she pricked her finger while making lace. The common name *bird's nest* comes from the tendency of the flower heads to curve upward, forming a basket.

Much smaller than today's cultivated carrot, the root was a common food in ancient Greece and Rome. Native to Asia, wild carrot is used in Traditional Chinese Medicine. When the plant was introduced into Britain during the sixteenth century, the flowers and leaves became popular hair accessories. The species name is derived from the Greek word *karoton*, meaning "carrot," and *Daucus* is the Latin name for the plant.[28]

Oil Description and Precautions

Steam distillation of the seeds produces a yellow to amber oil that has a thin to medium viscosity. It has an approximate shelf life of two to threes years or slightly longer. Avoid carrot seed essential oil during pregnancy and while breastfeeding.

28. Coombes, *Dictionary of Plant Names*, 70.

Blending for Scent

Carrot seed has an earthy, herbaceous, and slightly spicy scent. Some of the oils that blend well with it include bergamot, cedarwood, cinnamon leaf, geranium, ginger, lemon, lime, and mandarin.

Scent Group	Perfume Name	Initial Strength	Sun Sign
Herbaceous	Middle	Medium to strong	Virgo

Medicinal Remedies

This essential oil is used for arthritis, burns, corns and calluses, cuts and scrapes, dermatitis, eczema, edema, gout, indigestion, premenstrual syndrome (PMS), psoriasis, rashes, and sunburn.

Carrot seed's strong point is its ability to heal skin conditions, especially eczema, dermatitis, and psoriasis. Combine 6 to 10 drops of carrot seed with 2 tablespoons of jojoba carrier oil and apply several times a day to soothe these and other itchy rashes. For burns, add 2 drops of carrot seed and 1 drop of lavender or tea tree to a tablespoon of carrier oil. The combination of carrot and tea tree also works well for first aid on cuts and scrapes. When dealing with gout, arthritis, or general joint pain, combine 5 drops each of carrot seed and rosemary and 3 drops of juniper berry in an ounce of carrier oil for a warming massage.

Personal Care and Well-Being

Carrot seed is excellent for skin care, especially mature skin, because it restores elasticity and helps reduce wrinkles. Combining it with frankincense and neroli is particularly effective to revitalize the complexion. It also works well with geranium for skin care. To relieve an itchy scalp, add 2 to 3 drops of carrot seed to a teaspoon of olive oil and gently massage it in. Leave the oil on for about ten minutes before shampooing. Carrot seed is also appropriate to use on normal hair.

Getting the feet ready for sandals in the summer usually means dealing with calluses. Begin your regimen to get rid of this hard skin with a foot soak. Add 1 to 6 drops of carrot seed to a teaspoon of carrier oil and swish into a basin of warm water. When the water cools, wet a pumice stone and gently rub the callused area. Afterward, massage the area with the following treatment.

Carrot Seed Callus Treatment

1½ tablespoons cocoa butter, grated or shaved

1 tablespoon coconut oil

. . . .

10 drops carrot seed essential oil

8 drops lemon essential oil

Boil a little water in a saucepan and remove it from the heat. Place the butter and carrier oil in a jar in the water and stir until the butter melts. Remove the jar from the water, allow the mixture to cool to room temperature, then repeat the process. When it cools again, add the essential oils and mix thoroughly. Place it in the refrigerator for five or six hours. Allow the mixture to come to room temperature before using or storing.

The calming scent of carrot seed is an aid for lifting moods and coping with unexpected changes. For emotional support, diffuse 2 parts each of carrot seed and palmarosa and 1 part orange. When engaging in energy work, carrot seed activates the root and sacral chakras. It is an aid when praying for healing and in candle magic for attracting abundance.

For the Home
To maintain harmonious energy in your home, use carrot seed in a reed diffuser or feng shui salts. Carrot seed is particularly effective for balance after mediating fast-moving energy.

The Cedarwood Oils

Cedars are called *arbor vitae*, the "tree of life," not only because of their majestic stature but also because for thousands of years they provided many essentials of daily life. Although Virginia cedarwood is technically a juniper, it is commonly called *cedar* because of its scent.

❧ Cedarwood, Atlas ❧

BOTANICAL NAME: *Cedrus atlantica*

ALSO KNOWN AS: African cedar, Atlantic cedar, libanol oil, Moroccan cedarwood oil

Native to the Atlas Mountains of Algeria and Morocco, this tree reaches almost a hundred feet tall, with an elegant pyramid shape. Its genus name is Latin for *cedar*, and its species name means "of the Atlas Mountains." [29] This tree is a close cousin to the famous cedar of Lebanon (*C. libani*).

The ancient Egyptians used cedar oil in perfumes and cosmetics and the wood for ships and furniture. Throughout the ancient world, cedarwood was prized for building material because it repelled harmful insects. Cedar oil was used medicinally in the Middle East and in Tibet, where it was also used for temple incense. Today, cedarwood is popular as a fixative in perfumes and cosmetics and in household products, especially insect repellents.

---

29. Coombes, *Dictionary of Plant Names*, 50.

· · · · · · · ·

Oil Description and Precautions

The wood is steam-distilled, producing an oil that ranges from deep amber to yellow to orange. Atlas cedarwood has a medium viscosity and a slightly oily texture. It has an approximate shelf life of four to six years. Avoid using this oil during pregnancy; may cause skin irritation.

Blending for Scent

Atlas cedarwood has a warm, woody, and slightly spicy scent. Some of the oils that blend well with it include bergamot, chamomile, juniper berry, palmarosa, petitgrain, rosemary, and vetiver.

Scent Group	Perfume Note	Initial Strength	Sun Signs
Woody	Middle to base	Strong	Aries, Sagittarius, Taurus

Medicinal Remedies

Atlas cedarwood essential oil is used for acne, arthritis, athlete's foot, bronchitis, colds, coughs, dermatitis, eczema, and stress.

With anti-inflammatory properties, it relieves the pain and stiffness of arthritis. For massage, add 6 to 8 drops of cedarwood to a tablespoon of carrier oil. If you prefer a healing soak in the tub, combine 2 cups of Epsom or sea salt with 10 drops of cedarwood and 5 drops of cinnamon leaf or thyme.

Atlas cedarwood's antifungal properties relieve the itching that often occurs with fungal infections. Combine 6 drops of cedarwood and 3 drops of lemongrass in a tablespoon of carrier oil and gently apply to the area.

Personal Care and Well-Being

The astringent and antibacterial properties of cedarwood make it ideal for oily skin and blemishes. It is also good for oily hair and dandruff. Combine a drop each of cedarwood and clary sage in a teaspoon of carrier oil and use it to massage the scalp. Afterward, shampoo and rinse thoroughly. Cedarwood is also helpful when dealing with hair loss.

This essential oil is particularly good for calming anger and bringing emotions into balance. It aids in dealing with grief following the death of a loved one. To relieve tension and foster peace, diffuse 3 parts cedarwood and 1 part each of geranium and lemon. Cedarwood also fosters mental clarity.

For energy work, cedarwood activates and balances all of the chakras. Use it to purify an area when consecrating an altar or meditation space. When used in candle magic, cedarwood helps banish negativity, aids in finding justice, and attracts abundance. It also supports dream work.

· · · · · · ·

For the Home

Since ancient times, cedarwood chests have been used to protect clothing and linens. Today, sachets provide an easy way to employ the power of cedar wherever it is needed. Use a sachet to protect winter clothes when you put them away for the summer or to freshen a linen closet. The following recipe is enough for several 3 x 5-inch muslin bags. When the scent fades, refresh the sachets with 4 drops of cedarwood and 2 drops each of the other oils.

Moths Be Gone Cedarwood Sachets

1 teaspoon carrier oil or blend

15 drops cedarwood essential oil

8 drops bergamot essential oil

8 drops lavender essential oil

1 cup baking soda

Combine all the oils, stir in the baking soda, and mix thoroughly. Use a fork to break up any clumps. Let the mixture dry, then pour it into muslin bags.

For aromatic feng shui, place a cedarwood candle or jar of salts wherever you need to stimulate the energy of your home.

❧ Cedarwood, Virginia ❧

BOTANICAL NAME: *Juniperus virginiana*

ALSO KNOWN AS: American red cedarwood oil, Eastern red cedar, red cedar, Virginia juniper

Indigenous to thirty-seven states in the United States, Virginia cedarwood is the most widely distributed eastern conifer. It has dense horizontal branches and a pyramidal crown. Usually growing thirty to forty feet, it can sometimes reach as tall as ninety feet. Its genus name is Latin for *juniper*.[30]

Native Americans used many parts of the tree for medicinal purposes from coughs and colds to wounds and joint stiffness. In addition to making tea from the berries, early European settlers used them medicinally. Colonists used the wood for furniture, fencing, and boats. It is still a popular wood for cedar chests.

Oil Description and Precautions

The wood is steam-distilled, producing a colorless to pale yellow oil. It has a medium viscosity and a slightly oily texture. Its shelf life is approximately two to three years. This cedarwood is an abortifacient, so do not use during pregnancy; may cause skin irritation.

30. Coombes, *Dictionary of Plant Names*, 111.

• • • • • • •

Blending for Scent

Virginia cedarwood has a woody and sweetly balsamic scent. Some oils that blend well with this cedarwood include cinnamon leaf, citronella, cypress, frankincense, lavender, lemon, neroli, rose, and rosemary.

Scent Group	Perfume Note	Initial Strength	Sun Signs
Woody	Middle to base	Strong	Aries, Sagittarius, Taurus

Medicinal Remedies

Virginia cedarwood is used for acne, anxiety, arthritis, bronchitis, colds, coughs, eczema, psoriasis, rashes, sinus infection, stress, and warts.

With balsamic qualities, cedarwood eases the pain and stiffness of arthritis. Use it on its own or combine 5 drops of cedarwood, 3 drops of fir needle, and 4 drops of cypress with a tablespoon of carrier oil to massage away pain. This woody blend of oils also relieves the discomforts of bronchitis. Use 5 drops of cedarwood and 1 drop each of fir needle and pine in a quart of water for a steam inhalation.

Personal Care and Well-Being

Cedarwood helps keep the skin's oil production in check. Make an astringent with ¼ cup of chamomile tea, 1 tablespoon of witch hazel, and 16 to 18 drops of cedarwood. Shake well and apply to the face with a cotton ball. To help curb scalp oil, use 4 drops of cedarwood in a tablespoon of light carrier oil such as sweet almond. Massage it on the scalp for a few minutes, then shampoo and rinse well. Cedarwood also helps with itchy dandruff.

With its insect-repellent properties, cedarwood not only is useful for clothes chests and closets but also works well to spray on exposed arms and legs before heading outside in the summer. A drop of lavender can be added to the following recipe.

Cedarwood Insect Repellent

½ teaspoon carrier oil

3 drops cedarwood essential oil

2 ounces water

Combine the carrier and essential oils in a bottle with a fine spray nozzle. Add the water and shake well before each use.

To help balance moods, dispel anger, or release nervous tension, diffuse equal amounts of cedarwood and juniper berry. Use cedarwood to create a peaceful atmosphere or to ease sorrow

. . . .

when dealing with death. It also helps to focus the mind. For energy work, this cedarwood activates and balances all of the chakras.

Combine cedarwood with sandalwood to consecrate an altar or meditation space. When seeking justice, use cedarwood in candle magic. It can also be used to attract abundance and banish negative energy. Cedarwood supports dream work too.

For the Home

In addition to being an effective insect repellent against mosquitoes and moths, cedarwood is a scent that vermin, especially rats, dislike. Place several drops on cotton balls to scatter in areas where mice or rats may enter your home or garage. Be sure that pets and children cannot access the cotton balls. For aromatic feng shui, place a cedarwood candle or jar of salts wherever you need to stimulate energy.

The Chamomiles

Although German chamomile was sometimes considered a weed, both types of chamomile have been used interchangeably for a range of ailments since the time of the ancient Egyptians and Greeks. Medieval monks deemed chamomile "the plants' physician" because of the healthy effect it has on other garden plants.[31]

❧ Chamomile, German ❧

BOTANICAL NAME: *Matricaria recutita* syn. *M. chamomilla*
ALSO KNOWN AS: Blue chamomile, common chamomile, mayweed, wild chamomile

Growing two to three feet tall, German chamomile stands erect, with branching stems and feathery leaves. Its small daisy-like flowers have white petals and yellow centers. Although the flowers are less fragrant than those of Roman chamomile, the plant was used during the Middle Ages as a strewing herb on floors to combat pests and odor.

Oil Description and Precautions

Steam distillation of the flower heads produces a dark blue oil with a medium viscosity. It has an approximate shelf life of two to three years. Chamomile is an anti-allergenic for most people;

---

31. Staub, *75 Exceptional Herbs for Your Garden*, 48.

however, those with allergies to plants in the Asteraceae family should check for sensitivity before using it. German chamomile may cause dermatitis in some.

Blending for Scent

This chamomile has a warm and sweetly herbaceous scent. Some oils that blend well with it include frankincense, geranium, grapefruit, helichrysum, lavender, lemon, marjoram, neroli, patchouli, rosemary, tea tree, and ylang-ylang.

Scent Group	Perfume Note	Initial Strength	Sun Signs
Herbaceous	Middle to base	Medium to strong	Cancer, Leo

Medicinal Remedies

German chamomile is used for acne, anxiety, arthritis, boils, burns, chicken pox, chilblains, cuts and scrapes, dermatitis, earaches, eczema, hay fever, headaches, indigestion, inflammation, insect bites and stings, insomnia, menopausal discomforts, menstrual cramps, motion sickness, muscle aches and pains, nausea, poison ivy, premenstrual syndrome (PMS), psoriasis, rashes, sprains and strains, stress, and sunburn.

While the properties of both chamomile essential oils are almost identical and the two are frequently used interchangeably, German chamomile has stronger anti-inflammatory properties. It helps ease arthritis and general muscle aches and pains. It also helps relieve menstrual cramps.

Ease the Pain Chamomile Massage Oil

2 drops German chamomile essential oil

2 drops marjoram essential oil

1 drop thyme essential oil

1 tablespoon carrier oil or blend

Mix the essential oils together and combine with the carrier oil. Store any leftover oil in a bottle with a tight-fitting cap.

With its anti-allergenic and analgesic properties, German chamomile is particularly effective for bee stings. Combining it with lavender makes it even more potent. Use 2 drops each of chamomile and lavender in a teaspoon of carrier oil. This combination of essential oils also works well as first aid for burns. To help bring down swelling, apply ice to a sprain or strain, then combine 2 drops of chamomile with 1 drop of thyme in a teaspoon of carrier oil and gently massage the area.

• • • • • • •

For headache relief, place 5 or 6 drops of chamomile in a tablespoon of carrier oil and add it to a quart of cool water. Give the water a swish before soaking a washcloth in it. Place the cloth across the forehead from temple to temple. A warm compress with chamomile helps to soothe puffy, irritated eyes. For menopausal hot flashes, make a cool compress with chamomile, geranium, and/or clary sage.

Personal Care and Well-Being

Chamomile is suitable for all skin types, including sensitive. It is especially effective in a moisturizer to heal sun- or wind-damaged skin.

To release nervous tension and foster a peaceful atmosphere, diffuse 3 parts chamomile, 2 parts orange, and 1 part cedarwood. This combination of oils also helps subdue anger. For energy work, chamomile activates all of the chakras and brings them into alignment. Spiritually, use it at your altar to aid in sending healing prayers. For candle magic, chamomile attracts prosperity and luck, fosters love, and aids in achieving success. Also use it to support dream work.

For the Home

After stimulating or calming the energy in your home with other oils, use German chamomile to maintain balance. Try it in a room spray; just a quick spritz once or twice every other day can be effective.

❧ Chamomile, Roman ☙

BOTANICAL NAME: *Chamaemelum nobile* syn. *Anthemis nobilis*

ALSO KNOWN AS: English chamomile, garden chamomile, sweet chamomile, true chamomile

Usually less than nine inches tall, Roman chamomile is a spreading herb with stems that creep along the ground. It has feathery leaves and small daisy-like flowers with white petals and yellow centers. This plant's genus and common names were derived from the Greek words *chamai*, meaning "on the ground," and *melon*, "apple," which describes its scent.[32] German physician and botanist Joachim Camerarius (1534–1598) added the word *Roman* to its name when he discovered it growing just outside the city of Rome.[33]

Oil Description and Precautions

The flower heads are steam-distilled, producing a pale blue oil that turns slightly yellow with age. It has a thin viscosity and an approximate shelf life of two to three years. As with German chamomile, Roman chamomile is an anti-allergenic for most people; however, those with aller-

---

32. Coombes, *Dictionary of Plant Names*, 53.
33. Wheelwright, *Medicinal Plants and Their History*, 84.

gies to plants in the Asteraceae family should check for sensitivity before using. This essential oil may cause dermatitis in some.

Blending for Scent

Roman chamomile has a herbaceous and sweet apple-like scent. Some of the oils that blend well with it include bergamot, cypress, eucalyptus, geranium, grapefruit, lemon, myrrh, and palmarosa.

Scent Group	Perfume Note	Initial Strength	Sun Signs
Herbaceous	Middle	Strong	Cancer, Leo

Medicinal Remedies

Roman chamomile is used for acne, anxiety, arthritis, boils, burns, chilblains, cuts and scrapes, depression, dermatitis, earaches, eczema, fever, hay fever, headaches, indigestion, inflammation, insect bites and stings, insomnia, menopausal discomforts, menstrual cramps, migraines, motion sickness, muscle aches and pains, nausea, poison ivy, premenstrual syndrome (PMS), psoriasis, rashes, sore throat, sprains and strains, stress, sunburn, and tonsillitis.

A soothing bath with chamomile relieves the discomforts of psoriasis and eczema and helps heal the skin. Combine 15 to 20 drops of essential oil in an ounce of apricot kernel carrier oil to swish into the tub. To promote the healing of other rashes, use 2 drops of chamomile and 1 drop of helichrysum in a teaspoon of carrier oil and gently apply it to the area.

To treat boils, make a warm compress using 3 drops each of chamomile and tea tree in a tablespoon of carrier oil swished into a quart of water. Freshen the compress cloth frequently to keep it warm. Combine chamomile with an equal amount of spearmint in an inhaler or a few drops each in a tissue to quell nausea.

Personal Care and Well-Being

Like its cousin, Roman chamomile is also good for all skin types. For a cleansing facial steam, use 4 drops of chamomile and 2 drops each of lavender and myrrh in a quart of water. Follow this with a moisturizer of 1 or 2 drops of chamomile in a teaspoon of sweet almond carrier oil.

While chamomile is especially good for the complexion, don't forget the rest of your body. To use the chamomile chocolate bar in the following recipe, hold a section of it between your palms for a few moments; the warmth of your hands will melt the oils. Rub it on before or after a shower or bath.

Moisturizing Chamomile Chocolate Bars

6 tablespoons cocoa butter, grated or shaved

3 tablespoons carrier oil or blend

· · · · · · ·

8 drops vitamin E oil

½ teaspoon Roman chamomile essential oil

¼ teaspoon geranium essential oil

Boil a little water in a saucepan and remove it from the heat. Place the cocoa butter, carrier oil, and vitamin E in a jar and place it in the water. Stir until the butter melts. Remove the jar from the water and allow the mixture to cool to room temperature. Repeat the process, allow it to cool again, then add the essential oils. Pour the mixture into a candy bar mold and place in the fridge for five or six hours. Allow the bar to sit for a day before removing it from the mold. Break it into sections and store in a jar in a cool place.

To promote peaceful feelings and control anger, diffuse 2 parts chamomile and 1 part each of lavender and rose or palmarosa. This combination of oils will also help to soothe nervous tension. For help in getting a restful night's sleep, place a reed diffuser with chamomile on your bedside table.

For energy work, use chamomile to activate any individual chakra, or use it to bring all of them into balance. Use a little chamomile to help send healing prayers. For candle magic, chamomile helps to attract prosperity and luck, foster love, and achieve success. Also use this oil to support dream work.

For the Home

Place chamomile feng shui salts in a few areas around your house to keep the energy in balance. With its fresh apple scent, it is particularly effective in the kitchen.

☙ Cinnamon Leaf ❧

BOTANICAL NAME: *Cinnamomum zeylanicum* syn. *C. verum, Laurus cinnamomum*

ALSO KNOWN AS: Ceylon cinnamon, Madagascar cinnamon, true cinnamon

Native to parts of Southeast Asia, cinnamon is a tropical evergreen tree that grows to about fifty feet tall. It has shiny leathery leaves, yellow-white flowers, and bluish-white berries. The genus and common names were derived from the Greek *kinnamon* or *kinnamomon*, meaning "sweet wood," which in turn is thought to have come from the Malayan and Indonesian *kayamanis*, with the same meaning.[34] The people of Sri Lanka were the first to cultivate this tree.

Cinnamon has been one of the world's most important spices. It was a valuable commodity for the Phoenicians and Arabs in trade with the Egyptians, Greeks, and Romans. Like pepper,

---

34. Cumo, *Foods That Changed History*, 89.

cinnamon was one of the spices that spurred European traders to explore the world for new and faster routes to the Far East.

Oil Description and Precautions

The leaves are steam or water distilled, producing a yellow to brownish oil. It has a medium viscosity and a slightly oily texture. Cinnamon leaf has an approximate shelf life of two to three years or slightly longer. Avoid this essential oil during pregnancy; may cause skin irritation; use in moderation and in low concentrations.

Only information about oil from the cinnamon leaf is contained in this entry. The oil made from cinnamon bark is a dermal toxin and one of the most hazardous essential oils.

Blending for Scent

Cinnamon leaf oil has a warm, spicy scent. Some oils that blend well with it include cardamom, clove bud, ginger, grapefruit, lavender, lemon, orange, petitgrain, rosemary, and thyme.

Scent Group	Perfume Note	Initial Strength	Sun Signs
Spicy	Middle	Medium	Aries, Capricorn, Leo

Medicinal Remedies

Cinnamon leaf essential oil is used for arthritis, bronchitis, circulation, colds, coughs, depression, fever, flu, head lice, insect bites and stings, menstrual cramps, muscle aches and pains, scabies, stress, and warts.

To soothe the pain of bee stings, especially wasps, put a drop of cinnamon leaf in a teaspoon of carrier oil and gently apply to the site. Alternatively, make a cool compress by placing 2 or 3 drops in a tablespoon of carrier oil and adding it to a quart of cool water. To combat head lice, combine 2 drops of cinnamon leaf and 8 drops of tea tree in 2 tablespoons of carrier oil. Work it into the scalp and through the hair. Leave it on for about an hour, then shampoo and rinse thoroughly.

The antiseptic properties of cinnamon leaf help with coughs and colds. For a steam inhalation, combine 2 drops each of cinnamon, rosemary, and lemon in a quart of water. The disinfectant properties of cinnamon leaf will also help clean the air of a sickroom.

Well known as a warming spice, cinnamon essential oil can bring relief from arthritis. Combine 3 drops each of cinnamon leaf, coriander, and ginger and 2 drops of lemon in an ounce of carrier oil to massage away stiffness and pain.

Personal Care and Well-Being

Because cinnamon leaf can cause skin irritation, it is not used for personal care products; however, it is an aid for emotional support. To help maintain moods on an even keel, diffuse 1 part each of cinnamon and cardamom with 2 parts lavender. When you need clarity to focus on work or school, combine it with mandarin and rosemary. Cinnamon leaf also helps alleviate depression and nervous exhaustion.

For energy work, use cinnamon to activate the solar plexus, heart, and third eye chakras. Use it in the melted wax of a pillar candle for meditation and spiritual support. Cinnamon leaf can also be used to bless an altar or special space. In candle magic, it helps you find justice, attract luck, and reach your goals. It also enhances dream work.

For the Home

Bring the warm scent of cinnamon to your blankets or other linens for a cozy feeling in bed or when snuggling on the couch. Add a few drops of cinnamon leaf essential oil to a washcloth or dryer ball and toss it in the dryer with the blankets. Because essential oils can be flammable in certain conditions, use the dryer on a cool setting to fluff blankets and linens.

For aromatic feng shui, use cinnamon leaf to stimulate energy. Candles help set a special tone for the winter holiday season. When you don't want to leave them burning, a reed diffuser can continuously spread good cheer.

Cinnamon Winter Holiday Reed Diffuser

2 teaspoons essential oil blend using cinnamon leaf, clove bud, orange, and rosemary

¼ cup sunflower carrier oil

1 decorative jar

4–5 rattan reeds

Blend the essential oils in amounts that appeal to you, then combine them with the carrier oil. Pour the mixture into a jar and insert the reeds. Turn the reeds at least once a day to diffuse the scent.

✿ Citronella ✿

BOTANICAL NAME: *Cymbopogon nardus* syn. *Andropogon nardus*
ALSO KNOWN AS: Ceylon citronella, mosquito grass, nard grass, Sri Lanka citronella

Anyone who enjoys backyard cookouts is familiar with (and grateful for) citronella candles. The cultivated citronella plant is a descendant of the wild mana grass (*C. confertiflorus*) of Sri Lanka. With long, narrow leaf blades, it grows in clumps that can reach up to six feet wide and tall. Citronella is a cousin to lemongrass and palmarosa. The common name *citronella* was derived from the French word *citronnelle*, meaning "lemon liquor" or "lemon water" because of its scent.[35]

---

35. Barnhart, ed., *The Barnhart Concise Dictionary of Etymology*, 127.

For millennia, citronella was used medicinally in the Far East to treat a wide range of ailments. It was introduced into Europe in the nineteenth century for use as a room disinfectant and insect repellent to keep moths from making themselves at home in linen cupboards. Cats and rodents are not fond of it either. While the use of citronella waned during the early twentieth century, it has made a strong comeback since the chemical DDT was banned.

Oil Description and Precautions

Steam distillation of the leaves produces a yellow-brown oil. It has a thin viscosity and an approximate shelf life of two to three years. Avoid using citronella during pregnancy; may cause skin irritation; do not use on children under six years old.

It is important to note that another essential oil made from the Java citronella plant (*C. winterianus*) is available on the market. It is stronger and has different precautions.

Blending for Scent

Citronella has a fresh lemony sweet and slightly herbaceous scent. Some oils that blend well with it include bergamot, cedarwood, eucalyptus (lemon), geranium, lemon, orange, pine, sandalwood, and vetiver.

Scent Group	Perfume Note	Initial Strength	Sun Sign
Herbaceous	Top	Medium	Taurus

Medicinal Remedies

Citronella is used for anxiety, colds, depression, fever, flu, hay fever, head lice, headaches, inflammation, insect bites and stings, migraines, and stress.

The antiseptic and antibacterial properties of citronella help to ease cold and flu symptoms. For a steam inhalation, swish 3 drops of citronella and 1 drop each of pine and eucalyptus (blue) into a quart of water. To warm up in a therapeutic bath, use 10 drops of citronella, 6 drops of cedarwood, and 4 drops of peppermint in an ounce of carrier oil to add to the water. Diffuse citronella to freshen and clean the air of a sickroom.

Citronella in a warm foot soak can ease a pounding headache. While it may seem counterintuitive, drawing the blood lower in the body helps to relieve pressure in the head. Combine 2 drops each of citronella, lavender, and pine in a teaspoon of carrier oil and swish it into a basin for a foot soak. Citronella on its own in a footbath deodorizes sweaty feet by killing the bacteria that causes odor.

While it is best known as an insect repellent, citronella also soothes and heals insect bites and stings. Add 2 or 3 drops to a teaspoon of carrier oil and apply to the site.

Personal Care and Well-Being

To ward off insects before they bite, mix 4 drops of citronella in ½ teaspoon of carrier oil, then combine it with 2 ounces of water in a spray bottle. Shake well and spritz exposed skin before heading outside. Alternatively, use 2 drops each of citronella and cedarwood (Virginia).

If your skin and/or hair tend to be oily, the astringent properties of citronella are a good match because they help to reduce excess oil. Citronella, cypress, and tea tree make a good combo for oily skin. In addition to controlling oil, citronella also helps to condition hair. Used in the bath, it can help deal with excessive perspiration.

Diffuse 3 parts citronella with 2 parts bergamot and 1 part palmarosa to help focus the mind. This will also relieve mental fatigue. For energy work, use citronella to activate the sacral, heart, and throat chakras. In addition to grounding and centering energy for meditation or prayer, citronella can be used in candle magic to neutralize any form of negativity. It also helps to cleanse and lighten the aura.

For the Home

Place a jar of citronella feng shui salts wherever you need to calm the energy in your home. With antiseptic and antibacterial properties, citronella not only freshens the air but also disinfects it. Use citronella in a tealight diffuser on a picnic table to keep mosquitoes away.

Combine 15 drops each of citronella and lavender in a cup of baking soda to make moth-deterring sachets for your closets. Used to deodorize a carpet, citronella will also discourage fleas from hanging around. Because cats are especially sensitive to essential oils and do not like citronella, using it on carpet is not recommended if you have a feline in the house.

Citronella Carpet Cleaner

15 drops citronella essential oil

10 drops bergamot essential oil

5 drops cedarwood essential oil

8 ounces baking soda

Combine the essential oils, then mix thoroughly with the baking soda. Break up clumps with a fork. Lightly sprinkle the powder on a carpet. Let it sit for twenty to thirty minutes, then vacuum well.

Clary Sage
SEE *THE SAGE OILS*

❧ Clove Bud ❧

BOTANICAL NAME: *Syzygium aromaticum* syn. *Eugenia caryophyllata*

Native to Indonesia, the clove tree has a pyramidal shape and reaches forty to fifty feet in height. It has white fluffy flowers that grow in clusters and large bright green leaves. The familiar clove is a dried unopened flower bud.

Cloves were an early export commodity to China and India, where they were highly prized for culinary and medicinal purposes. By 176 CE, the Egyptians were enjoying them, and not much later, the Greeks and Romans were too.[36] Like other sought-after trade goods, clove was another spice that spurred European traders to explore the world for better routes to the East. Derived from either the French *clou* or the Latin *clavus*, both meaning "nail," an early Chinese name for cloves meant "sweet smelling nail." [37]

Oil Description and Precautions

Water or steam distillation of the flower buds produces a pale yellow oil. It has a medium viscosity and a slightly oily texture. Clove bud has an approximate shelf life of two to three years or slightly longer. Avoid this essential oil during pregnancy; may irritate the skin and mucus membranes; use in moderation.

Only information about oil from the clove bud is contained in this entry. Two other essential oils, one made from the leaves and another from the stems, are regarded as hazardous.

Blending for Scent

Clove bud essential oil has a sweet, spicy scent with a slightly fruity tinge. Some oils that blend well with it include basil, bergamot, chamomile, ginger, helichrysum, lavender, lemon, orange, palmarosa, and sandalwood.

Scent Group	Perfume Note	Initial Strength	Sun Signs
Spicy	Middle	Strong	Aries, Leo, Pisces, Scorpio, Sagittarius

Medicinal Remedies

Clove bud essential oil is used for anxiety, arthritis, asthma, athlete's foot, bronchitis, bruises, burns, chicken pox, colds, coughs, cuts and scrapes, flu, hay fever, lumbago, muscle aches and pains, nail fungus, nausea, shingles, sprains and strains, and stress.

36. Prance and Nesbitt, eds., *The Cultural History of Plants*, 161.

37. Weiss, *Spice Crops*, 106.

Like many of the pungent spices, clove bud helps relieve the respiratory discomforts associated with coughs, colds, and the flu. Its expectorant properties help to clear excess mucus. For relief on the go, combine 3 drops of clove and 4 drops each of orange and hyssop in an inhaler to take along. Take advantage of clove's antibacterial and antiseptic properties by using it in a diffuser to clean the air as a preventive measure during flu season. Use in small amounts and disperse it for brief intervals.

Clove bud can be used for several types of fungal infections and is particularly effective against stubborn nail fungus. Be sure to do a patch test first.

Clove Bud Knock Out Nail Fungus Treatment

3 drops carrier oil

1 drop clove bud essential oil

Combine the carrier and essential oils. Use a cotton swab to coat the nail and a small area of skin around it. Wait a few minutes, then cover with an adhesive bandage. Apply two or three times a day.

The antiviral properties of clove bud work well to quell the itching and numb the pain of shingles and chicken pox rashes. For shingles, combine 2 drops of clove bud with 4 drops of lemon balm in a tablespoon of carrier oil and apply gently. For chicken pox, combine it with lavender.

Just as the scent of clove in aromatherapy or cooking is warm and comforting, so too is its use in soothing painful joints and muscles. Make a massage blend using 2 drops each of clove bud and ginger and 4 drops of chamomile (German) in a tablespoon of carrier oil. This combination of oils also works well for a healing bath.

Personal Care and Well-Being

While clove bud is not used for skin and hair care, its comforting scent provides emotional support and promotes general well-being. It stimulates the mind, lifts the spirit, and aids concentration. For energy work, use clove bud to activate the root and solar plexus chakras.

For support during meditation and spiritual practices, place a drop of clove bud in the melted wax of a pillar candle. When used in candle magic, it banishes negativity and fosters happiness. It also attracts luck and aids in achieving success.

For the Home

Although the classic pomander (an orange studded with cloves) is mostly used for decorative purposes during the winter holidays, in the past it was an effective method for freshening the air and repelling insects. In lieu of making a pomander, diffuse 1 part clove bud with 2 parts each of bergamot and lemon.

• • • • • • • •

For battling mold and mildew, use clove bud and cedarwood with white vinegar. Pour ½ cup of vinegar into a spray bottle and add 3 or 4 drops each of clove and cedarwood essential oils. Shake gently and spray a little bit on the affected areas. Do not rinse. In addition to cutting the odor of vinegar, the essential oils in this spray also help kill fungus. Use clove bud feng shui salts or a few drops in the melted wax of a pillar candle to get energy moving.

❧ Coriander ❧

BOTANICAL NAME: *Coriandrum sativum*

ALSO KNOWN AS: Chinese parsley, cilantro, coriander seed, Italian parsley

This plant is known by two names: coriander and cilantro. Technically, coriander refers to the seeds and cilantro to the lower leaves. With erect, slender stems, this strongly aromatic herb grows about two feet tall. The golden brown ball-shaped seeds are less than ¼ inch in diameter. The genus and common names for the plant come from the Greek *koriandron*, which was derived from the word *koris*, meaning "bug," referring to the smell of the leaves and unripe seeds.[38]

With their use dating to the Sumerian and Babylonian civilizations, coriander seeds are one of the oldest and most highly prized food flavorings. They were used in Egypt and around the Mediterranean as early as 1500 BCE.[39] The Greeks and Romans used the seeds for medicinal and culinary purposes, as well as a flavoring for wine. Coriander was also used as an aphrodisiac. The Romans introduced the plant into Western Europe and Britain. Today, coriander is widely used as a flavoring in a range of foods and beverages, including several liqueurs.

Oil Description and Precautions
Steam-distilling the seeds produces a colorless to pale yellow oil with a medium viscosity. Coriander has an approximate shelf life of two to three years. Do not use this essential oil during pregnancy; use in moderation.

Blending for Scent
Coriander essential oil has a sweet, spicy, and slightly woody scent. Some oils that blend well with it include cardamom, cinnamon leaf, cypress, ginger, grapefruit, lemon, lemongrass, neroli, orange, petitgrain, pine, sandalwood, and ylang-ylang.

Scent Group	Perfume Note	Initial Strength	Sun Sign
Spicy	Middle	Medium	Aries

---

38. Quattrocchi, *CRC World Dictionary of Plant Names*, 616.

39. Chevallier, *The Encyclopedia of Medicinal Plants*, 193.

Medicinal Remedies

Coriander is used for anxiety, arthritis, circulation, colds, flu, gout, headaches, indigestion, menopausal discomforts, menstrual cramps, migraines, muscle aches and pains, nausea, premenstrual syndrome (PMS), and stress.

Coriander essential oil is an analgesic that eases muscle and joint pain. Combine 3 drops of coriander with 4 drops each of rosemary and lime in an ounce of carrier oil to create an effective massage blend that also reduces stress. Coriander and rosemary make a good combination for temporomandibular joint pain (TMJ). Be sure to mix a 1% dilution for use on the face.

A soak in the tub is a soothing and effective way to deal with stress or relieve a headache. Combine coriander with neroli and lavender to make bath salts that you will want to use as more than an ailment remedy.

Coriander Soothing Bath Salts

4 tablespoons carrier oil or blend

5 drops lavender essential oil

3 drops coriander essential oil

3 drops neroli essential oil

2 cups Epsom or sea salt

Mix the carrier and essential oils. Place the salt in a glass or ceramic bowl, add the oils, and mix thoroughly. Store in a jar with a tight-fitting lid.

Coriander is effective to quell nausea. Place a couple of drops in a tissue or combine a few drops of carrier oil and coriander in your palm. Rub your hands together, then cup them over your nose. This also helps relieve nasal congestion when you have a cold.

Personal Care and Well-Being

Coriander works well for oily skin. Make an astringent with ¼ cup of chamomile tea, 1 tablespoon of witch hazel, 3 drops of coriander, and 4 drops each of bergamot and clary sage. Combine everything in a bottle, shake well, and apply to the face with a cotton ball. Because it inhibits the growth of bacteria, coriander is also effective as a deodorant ingredient.

The scent of coriander is gentle and comforting, bringing a sense of happiness, fidelity, and well-being. It calms irritability and helps you recover from nervous exhaustion. Diffuse 2 parts coriander and 1 part each of bergamot and palmarosa to help maintain emotional balance, especially when dealing with unanticipated upheavals in your life. Coriander is also effective to stimulate the mind and stoke creativity.

For energy work, use coriander to activate the sacral, solar plexus, and heart chakras. Also use it to bless sacred space in your home. Coriander provides support to send healing prayers and instills a peaceful feeling. Use it to attract love into your life with candle magic.

For the Home

Wherever you sense sluggish energy in your home, place a jar of coriander feng shui salts in the area to get things moving. Alternatively, use a little bit in a diffuser.

❧ Cypress ❧

BOTANICAL NAME: *Cupressus sempervirens*

ALSO KNOWN AS: Common cypress, Italian cypress, Mediterranean cypress

Native to the eastern Mediterranean region, cypress is a conical-shaped evergreen with slender branches, scale-like needles, and round knobby cones that grow in clusters. In ancient times, this statuesque tree was highly valued for medicinal and religious purposes. Small pieces were burned as incense to clean the air after illness, as well as for spiritual purification. The Phoenicians were fond of the wood for shipbuilding.

For millennia, the cypress has been associated with life and death. Its Latin species name means "evergreen," which is a reference not only to the tree retaining its color all year long but also to the fact that it was a symbol of immortality.[40] Although there are numerous versions of a Greek myth concerning a young man named Cyparissus, the gist of the story is that he was heartbroken after accidentally killing a beloved tame stag. His grief was so great that he was transformed into a cypress tree, which was a symbol of sorrow. For centuries, this tree was planted in cemeteries as a symbol of remembrance.

Oil Description and Precautions

The needles and twigs are steam-distilled, producing an oil that is pale yellow to slightly olive green. It has a thin viscosity and an approximate shelf life of twelve to eighteen months. Avoid using cypress essential oil during pregnancy and when breastfeeding.

Blending for Scent

This oil has a woody, slightly nutty, and spicy scent. Some oils that blend well with cypress include cedarwood, chamomile, ginger, grapefruit, lavender, lemon, lemongrass, neroli, orange, pine, and sandalwood.

---

40. Coombes, *Dictionary of Plant Names*, 113.

• • • • • • •

Scent Group	Perfume Note	Initial Strength	Sun Signs
Woody	Middle to base	Medium	Aquarius, Capricorn, Pisces, Taurus, Virgo

Medicinal Remedies

Cypress is used for arthritis, asthma, bronchitis, bursitis, cellulite, circulation, colds, coughs, cuts and scrapes, edema, flu, hemorrhoids, menopausal discomforts, muscle aches and pains, poison ivy, premenstrual syndrome (PMS), stress, tendonitis, varicose veins, and whooping cough.

The antispasmodic properties of cypress are effective for dealing with coughs, including bronchitis and whooping cough. In a pinch during a cough attack, place 1 or 2 drops of cypress on a tissue. The following inhaler recipe is for bronchitis and general coughs associated with colds. For whooping cough, combine cypress with hyssop and rosemary.

Calm the Cough Cypress Inhaler Blend

7 drops cypress essential oil

3 drops frankincense essential oil

1 drop orange essential oil

Drip the oils onto the wick of an inhaler tube or into a small bottle. Inhale a couple of breaths as needed.

The inhaler blend combination of essential oils also works well for a steam inhalation. When dealing with asthma, check with your doctor before using essential oils. If you use a steam inhalation to relieve asthma, instead of tenting your head with a towel, use your hand to waft the steam toward your face.

The anti-inflammatory properties of cypress help to ease the pain of varicose veins. Combine 3 drops each of cypress, bergamot, and sage in a tablespoon of carrier oil. Swish the mixture into a quart of warm water to make a compress. These three essential oils also work well to massage varicose veins. Gently massage upward toward the heart to help move blood out of the legs.

Personal Care and Well-Being

The astringent properties of cypress make it effective for dealing with oily skin and hair. It also aids hair growth. Combine it with lemon and peppermint to make a skin toner. Cypress is an aid when dealing with excessive perspiration; use it in the bath or in a deodorant. This oil is particularly soothing when used as a foot soak for sweaty, tired feet.

· · · · · · · ·

The refreshing fragrance of cypress calms the mind, settles emotions, and relieves nervous tension. It helps with anger and irritability too. Cypress supports mental clarity and emotional balance and is particularly helpful when navigating life's transitions. For support during times of bereavement, diffuse 3 parts cypress, 2 parts rose (or palmarosa), and 1 part frankincense. Cypress used on its own promotes a peaceful atmosphere.

For energy work, use this oil to activate the solar plexus, heart, throat, and third eye chakras. Known as a purifier, cypress is effective to consecrate an altar or sacred space. Use it to ground and center energy for meditation and prayer. Place a few drops of cypress in a small bowl as an altar offering to honor loved ones who have passed. In candle magic, cypress can be used to banish any type of negativity and foster happiness. It is also an aid when seeking justice.

For the Home

Cypress is especially effective for slowing fast-moving energy and creating a calm atmosphere. Make a room spray with it and use a spritz or two wherever an energy adjustment is needed. Cypress is also an insect repellent.

℘ Elemi ℘

BOTANICAL NAME: *Canarium luzonicum*

ALSO KNOWN AS: Elemi canary tree, Manila elemi tree, pili tree

Reaching almost a hundred feet high, this cousin to frankincense and myrrh has dark oblong leaves and yellowish-white flowers. Indigenous to the Philippines and parts of Indonesia, elemi was known throughout the ancient world. Burned as incense, the pungent oleoresin was an important trade commodity. In later centuries, it was used for making varnish and inks. The common name *elemi* was derived from the Arabic *al-lāmī*, meaning "the resin," and referred to elemi and several other trees in the *Canarium* genus.[41] Although it has a few medicinal applications, elemi essential oil's most important use is for skin care.

Oil Description and Precautions

A colorless to very pale yellow oil is produced through steam distillation of the oleoresin. It has a thin viscosity and an approximate shelf life of two to three years. This essential oil may irritate sensitive skin.

Blending for Scent

Elemi has a slightly spicy lemony scent with a mild balsamic undertone. Some oils that blend well with it include cinnamon leaf, frankincense, lavender, myrrh, rosemary, and sage.

41. *Webster's II New College Dictionary* (2005), s.v. "elemi," 372.

Scent Group	Perfume Note	Initial Strength	Sun Sign
Spicy	Middle	Mild to medium	Pisces

Medicinal Remedies

Elemi is used for bronchitis, colds, coughs, cuts and scrapes, headaches, inflammation, rashes, scars, sinus infection, stress, and stretch marks.

To soothe headaches, especially when they are sinus-related, diffuse equal amounts of elemi, eucalyptus (blue), and thyme. The antiseptic properties of these oils will clean the air and help treat sinus infection. This combination also eases colds and coughs. With expectorant properties, elemi makes a good steam inhalation for coughs, including bronchitis.

To reduce the appearance of scars and stretch marks, moisturize them with 2 drops of elemi in a teaspoon of carrier oil. Rosehip seed and borage carrier oils are especially effective for this. For rashes, make a compress with 4 or 5 drops of elemi in a tablespoon of carrier oil, then swish it into a quart of cool water. After soaking a washcloth, gently place it on the rash. To soothe the discomfort of heat rash, use elemi in the bath. Combine 8 to 10 drops of elemi in an ounce of carrier oil to add to your bathwater.

Personal Care and Well-Being

Elemi is appropriate for all skin types. It normalizes dry and oily skin and is especially nourishing for mature complexions. It combats wrinkles and helps rejuvenate and tone the skin. For skin that is sun- or wind-damaged or dry, combine elemi with frankincense and carrot seed. For mature skin, combine it with lavender and neroli. In the following recipe, rosehip seed oil can be substituted for borage.

Elemi Nighttime Moisturizer

2 tablespoons cocoa butter, grated or shaved

3 tablespoons borage carrier oil

12 drops elemi essential oil

10 drops lavender essential oil

8 drops palmarosa essential oil

8 drops neroli essential oil

Boil a little water in a saucepan and remove it from the heat. Place the butter and carrier oil in a jar in the water and stir until the butter melts. Allow the mixture to cool to room temperature. Repeat the heating process, and when the mixture cools again, add the essential oils. Place the jar in the refrigerator for five or six hours. Allow it to warm to room temperature before using or storing.

The fresh scent of elemi calms nervous tension and relieves mental fatigue. Use it in a diffuser to help deal with negative emotions, balance moods, and lift spirits. It is also an aid for concentration when mental clarity is needed. Used lightly throughout the house, elemi can foster a sense of peace.

For energy work, elemi activates the root, third eye, and crown chakras. It is helpful for grounding and centering energy before meditation or prayer and for general spiritual practices. It can be instrumental in sending healing prayers to those in need. When used in candle magic, elemi helps remove negative energy or anything that you no longer need in your life.

For the Home
Use elemi in feng shui salts or a candle wherever you need to mediate and calm the energy flow. To foster peaceful energy in outdoor areas, combine a few drops of elemi and an ounce of water in a spray bottle to use on a porch or patio.

The Eucalyptus Oils

The genus and common names of these trees come from the Greek word *eukalypto*, meaning "covered" or "wrapped," which describes how the hanging seedpods almost cover the young flower buds.[42] Eucalyptuses are called *gum trees* in reference to the sticky gumlike substance that they secrete. In the nineteenth century, these trees were introduced from Australia into California, Southern Europe, and other areas around the world.[43] Eucalyptus oil is a powerful antiseptic and is familiar to most people for treating colds.

ஜ Eucalyptus, Blue ஒ

BOTANICAL NAME: *Eucalyptus globulus*

ALSO KNOWN AS: Fever tree, gum tree, southern blue gum

Absorbing great amounts of water, the extensive root systems of these trees were employed to rid areas of mosquito-infested wetlands throughout Australia. Their camphoraceous scent also aided the effort as an insect repellent. In its habitat, this tree can grow over three hundred feet tall, but in areas where it was introduced, it reaches only half that size. The smooth blue-gray bark peels off in large pieces on the upper trunk, exposing the creamy color underneath. This tree has narrow yellowish-green leaves and creamy white flowers.

---

42. Coombes, *Dictionary of Plant Names*, 87.
43. Chevallier, *The Encyclopedia of Medicinal Plants*, 94.

· · · · · · · ·

Oil Description and Precautions

Steam distillation of the leaves produces a colorless oil that yellows with age. It has a thin viscosity and an approximate shelf life of two to three years or slightly longer. This essential oil is toxic if taken internally; may cause skin irritation; not compatible with homeopathic treatment; use in moderation; do not use on children under six years old.

Blending for Scent

This essential oil's camphoraceous scent has a woody, earthy undertone. Some of the oils that blend well with it include chamomile, cypress, ginger, juniper berry, lavender, lemon, pine, rosemary, and tea tree.

Scent Group	Perfume Note	Initial Strength	Sun Signs
Woody	Middle to top	Very Strong	Cancer, Capricorn, Pisces, Taurus

Medicinal Remedies

This eucalyptus oil is used for arthritis, asthma, blisters, boils, bronchitis, burns, bursitis, chicken pox, circulation, cold sores, colds, coughs, cuts and scrapes, fever, flu, hay fever, head lice, headaches, insect bites and stings, lumbago, muscle aches and pains, sinus infection, sore throat, and sprains and strains.

Blue gum eucalyptus is an anti-parasitic that can be used to treat head lice and scabies. For head lice, mix 3 or 4 drops in a tablespoon of carrier oil and gently massage it on the scalp. Wrap a towel around your head and leave it on for half an hour. Shampoo and rinse thoroughly. For scabies, an ointment works well, especially when combined with other oils.

Eucalyptus Scabies Ointment

¼ ounce beeswax

4 tablespoons carrier oil or blend

10 drops eucalyptus (blue) essential oil

14 drops lavender essential oil

8 drops pine essential oil

Place the beeswax and carrier oil in a jar in a saucepan of water. Warm it over low heat, stirring until the wax melts. Remove it from the heat and allow the mixture to cool to room temperature before adding the essential oils. Adjust the consistency if necessary. Allow the mixture to cool thoroughly before using or storing.

For relief from hay fever, combine 1 drop each of eucalyptus, chamomile, and lemon balm in a teaspoon of carrier oil. Apply a small dab to pulse points on wrists and inner elbows and to the chest. To relieve and heal cold sores, place a drop each of eucalyptus and bergamot in a teaspoon of carrier oil and apply with a cotton swab.

Personal Care and Well-Being

When used for skin care, eucalyptus helps to tone and balance the complexion. Mildly astringent, it reduces excess oil. It also works well as a facial steam for oily skin to unclog and clean pores. Eucalyptus helps to control dandruff and can be used on its own for a deodorant or combined with lavender and peppermint.

Emotionally, eucalyptus provides support when dealing with grief and helps to restore a sense of well-being. When you need emotional space, diffuse 3 parts eucalyptus, 2 parts lemon, and 1 part basil. Eucalyptus is also an aid for lifting fatigue and mental exhaustion.

For energy work, use eucalyptus to activate the heart chakra. Use it on your altar when praying for healing. This eucalyptus oil attracts happiness when used in candle magic. It also supports dream work and past-life work.

For the Home

Eucalyptus is a classic insect repellent. Use it in candles and diffusers to deter bugs in your home. For aromatic feng shui, use it to stimulate and move energy.

ꙮ Eucalyptus, Lemon ꙮ

BOTANICAL NAME: *Eucalyptus citriodora* syn. *E. maculata* var. *citriodora, Corymbia citriodora*

ALSO KNOWN AS: Lemon-scented gum tree, spotted gum

This eucalyptus species grows to about a hundred feet tall and has narrow tapering leaves. Its pale, slightly mottled bark sheds in curling flakes, giving the trunk a mottled or spotted appearance. With a species name meaning "lemon-scented," the oil of this tree has been widely used to perfume linen closets, as well as protect the contents against insects. Regarded as more elegant than other species of eucalyptus trees, it is frequently used as an ornamental plant.

Oil Description and Precautions

Steam distillation of the leaves and twigs produces a colorless or pale yellow oil with a thin viscosity. It has an approximate shelf life of two to three years or slightly longer. This essential oil is toxic if taken internally; may cause skin irritation; not compatible with homeopathic treatment; use in moderation.

Blending for Scent

This eucalyptus oil has a lemony citronella-like scent. Some oils that blend well with it include basil, black pepper, clary sage, clove bud, geranium, ginger, lavender, marjoram, orange, pine, ravintsara, tea tree, thyme, and vetiver.

Scent Group	Perfume Note	Initial Strength	Sun Signs
Citrus	Middle to top	Medium	Cancer, Capricorn, Pisces, Taurus

Medicinal Remedies

Lemon eucalyptus oil is used for asthma, athlete's foot, chicken pox, cold sores, colds, cuts and scrapes, fever, insect bites and stings, laryngitis, nail fungus, sinus infection, and sore throat.

While both eucalyptus essential oils help bring down a fever, lemon eucalyptus is a little more cooling than the blue gum. Make a compress using 5 or 6 drops in a tablespoon of carrier oil and add it to a quart of cool water. Give it a good swish before soaking a washcloth and applying.

The antiseptic and bactericidal properties of lemon eucalyptus make it a good first aid treatment for cuts, scrapes, and insect bites. Combine a drop or two in a teaspoon of carrier oil and gently apply. It will also help relieve the itching of athlete's foot. For extra power in soothing the feet, use 1 drop each of lemon eucalyptus and manuka.

Personal Care and Well-Being

Like other citrusy essential oils, lemon eucalyptus is a boon to oily skin, helping to reduce and regulate oils. It is also effective for treating pimple outbreaks. Use 1 or 2 drops in a teaspoon of apricot kernel or peach kernel carrier oil and apply with a cotton swab. Lemon eucalyptus is an effective deodorant and helps treat dandruff.

This oil helps you to deal with mood swings, cools anger, and brings emotions into balance. It is also effective to clear and focus the mind. To foster a sense of well-being, diffuse 2 parts lemon eucalyptus with 1 part each of cedarwood and marjoram.

Use this oil on the heart center to activate this chakra and on your altar to help when sending healing prayers. In candle magic, it can be used to attract happiness. Lemon eucalyptus also supports dream work and past-life work.

For the Home

Traditionally used as scent and insect repellent for linen cupboards, lemon eucalyptus is the only essential oil on the Environmental Protection Agency's (EPA) list of registered insect repellents for mosquitoes. It is also effective against cockroaches and silverfish, which can cause significant damage. Moths don't like lemon eucalyptus either. The vinegar in the following recipe also acts as a deterrent to some insects.

Eucalyptus Bug Out Spray

¼ cup white vinegar

¼ cup water

20 drops eucalyptus (lemon) essential oil

10 drops peppermint essential oil

10 drops lavender essential oil

10 drops tea tree essential oil

5 drops rosemary essential oil

Combine all the ingredients in a spray bottle. Shake well before each use.

To deter moths and other creepy-crawlies in linen and clothes closets, make sachets with 1 cup of baking soda, 15 drops of lemon eucalyptus, 10 drops of lavender, and 5 drops of peppermint.

To get the energy in your home moving, place lemon eucalyptus feng shui salts in any area where it feels sluggish. Burning a candle with this eucalyptus will also help.

᷒ Fennel, Sweet ᷒

BOTANICAL NAME: *Foeniculum vulgare* var. *dulce* syn. *F. dulce, F. vulgare, F. officinale*

ALSO KNOWN AS: French fennel, garden fennel, Roman fennel

Native to the Mediterranean region, fennel has a bulbous base, feathery leaves, and umbels of yellow flowers. It can reach five to six feet in height. Fennel's use for culinary and medicinal purposes dates to ancient times in China, India, and Egypt. The Greeks and Romans also used this plant for a wide range of ailments. Meaning "little hay" and referring to its scent, fennel's genus name was derived from the Latin word *foenum*, meaning "hay." [44] During the Middle Ages, this name evolved, becoming *fenkel* and eventually *fennill*. Medieval herbalists Nicholas Culpeper and John Gerard (1545–1612) sung its praises and recommended fennel for a range of ailments.

Oil Description and Precautions

Steam distillation of the seeds produces a colorless to pale yellow oil. It has a thin viscosity and an approximate shelf life of two to three years. Avoid this essential oil during pregnancy and

44. Weiss, *Spice Crops*, 285.

while breastfeeding; avoid if you have epilepsy or another seizure disorder; may cause sensitization; use in moderation; should not be used on children under six years old.

Fennel is a plant where the common name is as important as the botanical one, because *Foeniculum vulgare* and *F. officinale* are used for both sweet and bitter fennel. Although bitter fennel is grown as a vegetable, essential oil made from that plant is toxic and should never be used on the skin.

Blending for Scent

This essential oil has a spicy and sweetly anise-like scent. Some oils that blend well with it include bergamot, black pepper, cardamom, cypress, fir needle, geranium, juniper berry, lavender, mandarin, niaouli, rose, rosemary, and ylang-ylang.

Scent Group	Perfume Note	Initial Strength	Sun Signs
Spicy	Top	Medium	Aries, Gemini, Virgo

Medicinal Remedies

Fennel is used for arthritis, asthma, bronchitis, bruises, cellulite, constipation, coughs, edema, indigestion, inflammation, menopausal discomforts, nausea, premenstrual syndrome (PMS), and varicose veins.

When used for massage, fennel helps to decrease cellulite and reduce the swelling associated with edema. It also helps tone the skin. Use 12 to 14 drops in an ounce of carrier oil or try the following soothing blend.

Fennel Cellulite and Edema Massage Blend

3 tablespoons carrier oil or blend

6 drops fennel essential oil

8 drops cypress essential oil

6 drops geranium essential oil

Combine the oils and mix well. Store any leftover oil in a bottle with a tight-fitting cap.

A similar recipe made with 6 drops of fennel, 8 drops of lemon, and 6 drops of rosemary can be used to relieve the pain of varicose veins. To help ease constipation, use 6 to 8 drops of fennel in a tablespoon of carrier oil to massage the abdomen.

Fennel's antiseptic properties make it effective as a steam inhalation to relieve nasal congestion and reduce excess mucus. It also helps soothe coughs. To quell nausea, use the easy vapors method (from chapter 8) with 1 drop of fennel in a cup of steaming water.

Personal Care and Well-Being

Fennel is an aid for oily skin. To make an astringent, brew a cup of chamomile tea, and use 4 tablespoons of it with 1 teaspoon of witch hazel, 5 drops of fennel, and 6 drops of juniper berry. This mixture also brightens a dull complexion. Because it helps restore moisture and elasticity, fennel is helpful for mature skin. Make a basic moisturizer with 4 tablespoons of rosehip seed or jojoba carrier oil (or a blend of both), 3 drops of fennel, 5 drops of geranium, and 4 drops of frankincense. To reduce puffiness around the eyes, use fennel in a cool compress.

This oil is an aid for dealing with emotions and moods by fostering a sense of calmness and security. It provides support when initiating changes. To unblock emotions and energy, diffuse fennel with equal amounts of lemon and juniper berry. When working with the chakras, fennel activates the sacral and throat energy centers. For spiritual practices, fennel clears energy and can be used to consecrate an altar or sacred space. Use it in candle magic to draw love into your life.

For the Home

For aromatic feng shui, use fennel in a room spray wherever the energy feels sluggish. A candle made with fennel essential oil, even unlit, can stimulate energy.

✐ Fir Needle ✐

BOTANICAL NAME: *Abies alba* syn. *A. pectinata*
ALSO KNOWN AS: European silver fir, silver fir needle, white fir, white spruce

Native to the mountainous regions of Central and Southern Europe, fir was highly prized for its high-quality softwood timber. Like other firs, it is a source of turpentine. Growing in mixed forests, silver fir usually reaches between eighty and a hundred feet tall. Its needles are a shiny dark green with a lighter silvery color underneath. Young trees have a conical shape but become more columnar as they age. *Abies* is the classic Latin name for the tree, and *alba*, "white," refers to the bark of older trees.[45] The scent of this fir is widely used for fragrance in a range of commercial products.

Oil Description and Precautions

Needles and young twigs are steam-distilled, producing a colorless to pale yellow oil. It has a thin viscosity and a slightly oily texture. This essential oil has an approximate shelf life of nine to twelve months. Fir needle may cause skin irritation.

45. Coombes, *Dictionary of Plant Names*, 15.

· · · · · · ·

It is important to note that the information provided here only covers the essential oil from the silver fir (*A. alba*). Oils made from the balsam fir (*A. balsamea*) and hemlock spruce (*Tsuga canadensis*) are also called *fir needle*.

Blending for Scent

This essential oil has an earthy, woody, and slightly sweet balsamic scent. Some oils that blend well with fir needle include cedarwood, cypress, juniper berry, lavender, lemon, marjoram, orange, peppermint, pine, rosemary, and spearmint.

Scent Group	Perfume Note	Initial Strength	Sun Sign
Woody	Middle	Medium	Aries

Medicinal Remedies

Essential oil from the silver fir is used for arthritis, bronchitis, colds, coughs, fever, flu, muscle aches and pains, sinus infection, and stress.

Fir needle oil excels in treating coughs because of its strong antitussive and expectorant properties. Use it with other evergreen tree oils to soothe and relieve chest and nasal congestion. A salve can be used as a chest rub, or take it with you in a small jar to use as an inhaler. This combination of essential oils also makes an effective steam inhalation.

Fir Forest Cough and Cold Relief Salve

¼ ounce beeswax

3 tablespoons carrier oil or blend

9 drops fir needle essential oil

6 drops cypress essential oil

4 drops cedarwood essential oil

3 drops pine essential oil

Place the beeswax and carrier oil in a jar in a saucepan of water. Warm it over low heat, stirring until the wax melts. Remove it from the heat and allow the mixture to cool to room temperature before stirring in the essential oils. Adjust the consistency if necessary. Let it cool completely before using or storing.

To bring relief to sore muscles after hard work or active sports, combine 3 drops each of fir needle and marjoram in a tablespoon of carrier oil. The warming analgesic properties of fir are especially helpful for arthritis. Boost the effectiveness by combining 3 drops of it with 4 drops of rosemary and 1 drop of black pepper in a tablespoon of carrier oil.

• • • • • • • •

Personal Care and Well-Being

Because of its potential to irritate the skin, fir needle is usually not included in personal care preparations that are used frequently. The refreshing scent of fir needle aids in balancing emotions, especially when experiencing the ups and downs of coping with changes. Diffuse it with equal amounts of lemon and spearmint for emotional support and for help in lifting and balancing moods. Use fir needle with palmarosa to diminish mental fatigue and nervous tension. When dealing with grief, use 5 drops each of fir needle and cypress in an inhaler for support, as needed.

When used with lavender, fir needle can instill a deep sense of peace. It also supports meditation and spiritual practices. Use fir needle on its own to ground and center energy before praying, especially for healing. For energy work, this oil activates the root, sacral, throat, and crown chakras. It can be used in candle magic to attract abundance and prosperity and foster happiness.

For the Home

When used in a diffuser, fir needle cleans and deodorizes the air. In addition, its fresh scent creates a warm and welcoming environment. Use it for aromatic feng shui to stimulate energy wherever it feels bogged down and heavy.

Frankincense

BOTANICAL NAME: *Boswellia carteri*

ALSO KNOWN AS: Olibanum

Originating in the Red Sea region, this small shrubby tree has dense foliage and pale pink flowers. The name *frankincense* dates to the tenth-century French words *frank*, meaning "genuine," and *encens*, "incense," in reference to it being a high-quality incense.[46] The Latin name *olibanum* comes from the Arabic, *al-lubān*, meaning "milk," alluding to the appearance of the resin before it hardens after exposure to air.[47]

Believed to deepen the spiritual experience, frankincense was commonly burned in temples in China and India. It was also used medicinally. In addition to these purposes, the Egyptians valued frankincense for use in cosmetics and skin care. The tree was so highly prized that Queen Hatshepsut (reigned c. 1479–1458 BCE) had several transported to Egypt for her gardens.

Oil Description and Precautions

The oleoresin is steam-distilled, producing a pale yellow or greenish oil with a thin viscosity. It has an approximate shelf life of twelve to eighteen months. Avoid using this essential oil during pregnancy.

---

46. Barnhart, ed., *The Barnhart Concise Dictionary of Etymology*, 298.
47. Rodd and Stackhouse, *Trees: A Visual Guide*, 134.

Blending for Scent

Frankincense has a richly resinous and woody scent. Some oils that blend well with it include bergamot, black pepper, cypress, geranium, grapefruit, lavender, lemon, myrrh, orange, palma-rosa, sandalwood, vetiver, and ylang-ylang.

Scent Group	Perfume Note	Initial Strength	Sun Signs
Resinous	Base	Medium to strong	Aquarius, Aries, Leo, Sagittarius

Medicinal Remedies

Frankincense essential oil is used for anxiety, asthma, boils, bronchitis, colds, coughs, cuts and scrapes, flu, hemorrhoids, inflammation, laryngitis, poison ivy, premenstrual syndrome (PMS), scars, stress, and stretch marks.

The antiseptic properties of frankincense aid in healing minor cuts and scrapes. To treat a boil, use 2 drops of frankincense and 3 drops of lavender in a quart of warm water to make a compress. To soothe coughs and colds, combine equal amounts of frankincense and peppermint for a steam inhalation.

As an anti-inflammatory, frankincense helps relieve the discomfort of hemorrhoids. Combine 2 teaspoons of carrier oil with 2 drops each of frankincense, cypress, and geranium. Apply a few drops with a moistened tissue. The anti-inflammatory properties also help soothe the itching of poison ivy. Mix 4 drops of frankincense in ½ teaspoon of carrier oil and combine it with 2 ounces of water in a spray bottle. Shake well before each use. As an alternative, equal amounts of frankincense and helichrysum can be used.

Personal Care and Well-Being

For millennia, frankincense has been famous for its use in skin care. It is particularly rejuvenating for dry skin and helps tone mature complexions. Using it in a facial mask helps remove dirt from the pores and keep moisture in the skin.

Frankincense Fresh Face Mask

2 tablespoons white kaolin clay or oat flour

1 tablespoon yogurt or honey (or just enough to make a paste)

3 drops frankincense essential oil

2 drops elemi essential oil

2 drops carrot seed essential oil

Place the clay or oat flour in a bowl. Combine a little yogurt or honey with the essential oils, then mix thoroughly with the dry ingredient. Apply the paste close to the hairline, lips, and eyes. Just as it begins to dry, rinse thoroughly with warm water. Follow with a moisturizer.

To soothe puffy eyes, use equal amounts of frankincense and chamomile (Roman) to make a cool compress. For spider veins, combine a drop each of geranium and frankincense in a teaspoon of carrier oil and gently massage.

Frankincense is ideal for balancing moods, lifting spirits, and dealing with emotional turmoil, especially during transitions. Diffuse it on its own or combine 3 parts frankincense, 2 parts cedarwood, and 1 part mandarin. Frankincense also helps reduce nervous tension and foster mental clarity.

For meditation, frankincense is known to deepen the breath, which calms the emotions and focuses energy. Use it to activate any chakra individually or to bring them all into alignment. Place a drop each of frankincense, lavender, and bergamot in the melted wax of a pillar candle for meditation and spiritual support. Use frankincense on its own to consecrate sacred space or express gratitude. It can be instrumental when calling on angelic help or praying for healing.

In candle magic, use frankincense to remove negativity, foster happiness, or invite love into your life. It's also helpful when striving for success or seeking justice. Frankincense supports dream and past-life work.

For the Home

For aromatic feng shui, place frankincense salts or a candle wherever you need to balance the energy. This is particularly effective after calming or stimulating the energy flow.

❧ Geranium ❧

BOTANICAL NAMES: *Pelargonium roseum, P. capitatum × radens, P. cv. 'Rosé'*
ALSO KNOWN AS: Attar of rose geranium, bourbon geranium, geranium rosat, rose geranium, rose-scented geranium

Rose geranium presents a conundrum. First, it is not the familiar garden plant most of us know as a geranium. In fact, a great deal of uncertainty surrounds the exact botanical identification of geraniums. What is commonly referred to as a geranium is a pelargonium. *Geranium* and *Pelargonium* are names of genera in the Geraniaceae family. That's the easy part.

Confusion about these plants dates back several hundred years. In a craze for pelargoniums, so many hybrids were developed that they became indistinguishable. Compounding the problem is that different names were frequently given to a plant without reference to synonyms, and sometimes a name was given to several plants. In a few cases, hybrids were not named to distinguish them from their parent plants and some names lacked any botanical meaning. It's no wonder that confusion persists today.

Geranium essential oil is produced from two main hybrid species groups. The first group of hybrids is a cross between *P. capitatum* and *P. radens* (syn. *P. radula*). The second is between *P. capitatum* and *P. graveolens* (syn. *P.* × *asperum*). Rose-scented hybrids come from the first group.

Before the advent of chemically engineered scents, these plants were extremely important to the perfume industry because they were a less expensive alternative to roses. At one time, the island of Réunion in the Indian Ocean was the center of the rose geranium universe. In fact, for a time the name *rose geranium* was used only for plants cultivated there. The island's former name of Bourbon is also used in the name of some cultivars and essential oils.

Oil Description and Precautions

Steam distillation of the entire plant produces a greenish oil with a thin viscosity. It has an approximate shelf life of two to three years. Avoid using this essential oil during pregnancy; do not use on children under six years old; may cause sensitization.

Blending for Scent

This oil has a rosy, sweet, and somewhat minty scent. Some oils that blend well with geranium includes bergamot, carrot seed, clary sage, grapefruit, helichrysum, juniper berry, lavender, lemon balm, neroli, orange, petitgrain, rosemary, and sandalwood.

Scent Group	Perfume Note	Initial Strength	Sun Signs
Floral	Middle	Medium	Aries, Cancer

Medicinal Remedies

Geranium essential oil is used for acne, anxiety, bruises, burns, cellulite, circulation, cuts and scrapes, depression, dermatitis, eczema, edema, head lice, hemorrhoids, jet lag, menopausal discomforts, premenstrual syndrome (PMS), ringworm, shingles, sore throat, stress, sunburn, and tonsillitis.

Whether you have a burn from the kitchen or from fun in the sun, geranium helps soothe and heal the damage, especially when combined with aloe gel. Whip up a batch to keep on hand for quick first aid treatment.

Geranium and Lavender Burn Gel

2 tablespoons aloe gel

5 drops geranium essential oil

5 drops lavender essential oil

Combine all ingredients and mix well. Store in a jar with a tight-fitting lid.

To heal dermatitis and eczema, mix 1 drop each of geranium and juniper berry in a teaspoon of sweet almond carrier oil and apply gently. When dealing with menopausal or premenstrual issues, diffuse geranium with equal amounts of lavender and clary sage. For a sore throat, make a steam inhalation using 3 drops each of geranium and hyssop.

Personal Care and Well-Being

Cleansing and refreshing, geranium helps balance the skin's oil, whether you have a dry, mature, or oily complexion. For a quick moisturizer, combine a tablespoon of sweet almond carrier oil with 2 drops of geranium and 1 drop each of frankincense and chamomile. Substitute 1 drop each of bergamot and juniper berry for oily skin. Geranium also helps to combat wrinkles.

This essential oil comes to the rescue for dry hair and dandruff. Mix 2 drops each of geranium and myrrh in a tablespoon of coconut oil. Massage into the scalp and through the hair, then shampoo and rinse well. It can be used for normal hair too, and works well when used in a deodorant.

When dealing with any type of sorrow, geranium provides emotional support and restores a sense of well-being. Diffuse 2 parts each of geranium and grapefruit and 1 part ylang-ylang to calm nervous tension and foster a sense of peace. Geranium also helps to clear and focus the mind.

For energy work, geranium activates the solar plexus, heart, throat, and crown chakras. Use it when meditating and when praying for healing. It is effective for clearing the energy of meditation or sacred space. Geranium can be used in candle magic to attract love, happiness, and luck. Also use it for support in reaching goals.

For the Home

Geranium works well as an air freshener and goes nicely with lavender and mandarin. Diffuse geranium wherever you need to slow down fast-moving energy and bring it into balance.

✎ Ginger ✎

BOTANICAL NAME: *Zingiber officinale*

ALSO KNOWN AS: Common ginger, Jamaica ginger

The genus and common names for ginger evolved from the Latin word *zingiber*, which was derived from the Sanskrit *singabera*, meaning "horn-shaped."[48] This refers to the rhizomes

---

48. Foster and Johnson, *National Geographic Desk Reference to Nature's Medicine*, 180.

(roots), which resemble horns or antlers. Originating in southern Asia, this plant has reed-like stalks, spear-shaped leaves, and spikes of yellow or white flowers.

Ginger has been used for culinary and medicinal purposes in China and India for thousands of years. It was also used as an aphrodisiac. The Greeks and Romans imported ginger into Europe, where it remained a highly prized commodity through the Middle Ages. The Spanish introduced it into the West Indies and South America. Early European settlers in the United States used ginger to make what they called *small beer*, which resulted in ginger beer and ginger ale.

Oil Description and Precautions

A pale yellow, amber, or greenish oil is produced by steam distillation of the rhizomes. It has a thin viscosity and an approximate shelf life of two to three years. Ginger essential oil may cause skin irritation or sensitization; it is slightly phototoxic.

Blending for Scent

The scent of this oil is spicy, woody, and rich. Ginger blends well with cedarwood, clove bud, eucalyptus, geranium, grapefruit, lemon, lime, mandarin, neroli, palmarosa, patchouli, rose, vetiver, and ylang-ylang.

Scent Group	Perfume Note	Initial Strength	Sun Signs
Spicy	Middle to base	Strong to very strong	Aries, Leo, Scorpio, Sagittarius

Medicinal Remedies

Ginger essential oil is used for arthritis, bursitis, circulation, colds, constipation, coughs, depression, fever, flu, hangover, indigestion, jet lag, menstrual cramps, motion sickness, muscle aches and pains, nausea, seasonal affective disorder (SAD), sinus infection, sore throat, sprains and strains, and vertigo.

The antitussive and expectorant properties of ginger help to clear chest and nasal congestion. Diffuse 2 parts ginger and 1 part each of orange and frankincense to help fight off colds or ease symptoms if you catch one. Ginger's antispasmodic properties alleviate coughing. To relieve sinus infection, make a steam inhalation with 2 drops each of ginger, eucalyptus, and thyme.

Analgesic and warming, ginger relieves the pain and stiffness of arthritis. Combine 3 drops of ginger and 2 drops each of fir needle and rosemary in a tablespoon of carrier oil for a soothing massage.

Take an inhaler along when traveling to relieve motion sickness. Use 10 to 12 drops of ginger on its own or 6 drops of ginger and 5 drops of peppermint. This combination also helps to recover from jet lag or a hangover.

Personal Care and Well-Being

To relieve nervous exhaustion and mental fatigue, take time to relax while diffusing 2 parts ginger and 1 part each of lavender and peppermint. The warming glow of ginger-scented candles fosters an atmosphere of peace and well-being. (Read the full details about candle making in chapter 13.) The following recipe makes 3 to 4 tealight candles.

Brighter Day Ginger Candles

2 teaspoons blend of ginger, mandarin, and cedarwood (Virginia) essential oils

1 ounce beeswax

2 teaspoons coconut oil

Mix the essential oils together and adjust the amounts to get a scent balance you like. Place a glass measuring cup containing the wax and coconut oil in a saucepan of water and warm over low heat. Stir continuously until the wax melts, then remove it from the heat. Dip the bottom of the wick tabs in the wax and set one in the bottom of each tealight cup. Allow the mixture to cool. While it is still liquid, mix in the essential oils. Set the measuring cup in the pan of hot water for a minute if the essential oil congeals in the wax. Pour the wax into the tealight cups. When the candles are cool, trim the wicks. Give them a couple of days to set before using.

For help in grounding and centering your energy for meditation or prayer, combine ginger with geranium and mandarin in a diffuser or the melted wax of a pillar candle. Use ginger on its own to activate the root, sacral, solar plexus, and heart chakras. To attract abundance and prosperity into your life, use ginger in candle magic. It also fosters love.

For the Home

To freshen the air in your home, diffuse 3 parts mandarin, 2 parts neroli, and 1 part ginger. This combination also works well as a carpet deodorizer. For aromatic feng shui, use ginger to stimulate energy.

๛ Grapefruit ๛

Botanical name: *Citrus × paradisi*

Grapefruit is a natural hybrid of the pomelo (*C. maxima*) and sweet (*C. sinensis*) oranges that originated in the West Indies. The oranges were imported there from Southeast Asia in the late seventeenth century. The name *paradisi* was derived from the Latin word *paradisus* and the Greek word *parádeisos*, meaning "paradise." [49] Reaching about thirty feet tall, this tree has dense glossy foliage

---

49. Small, *Top 100 Food Plants*, 276.

and large white flowers. Growing in clusters, the small young fruit is green and has a slight resemblance to grapes.

Oil Description and Precautions

Cold-pressing the entire fruit produces a yellow or greenish oil with a thin viscosity. Although most citrus oils have an approximate shelf life of twelve to eighteen months, grapefruit is on the short end of the scale. This essential oil may cause skin irritation; it is phototoxic; avoid if taking medication not compatible with grapefruit.

Blending for Scent

This oil has a sweet, citrusy scent. Some oils that blend well with grapefruit include cardamom, chamomile (Roman), coriander, cypress, juniper berry, lemon, neroli, orange, palmarosa, and spearmint.

Scent Group	Perfume Note	Initial Strength	Sun Signs
Citrus	Middle to top	Strong	Gemini, Virgo

Medicinal Remedies

This essential oil is used for acne, cellulite, circulation, colds, depression, flu, hangover, headaches, nausea, premenstrual syndrome (PMS), seasonal affective disorder (SAD), stress, and varicose veins.

Grapefruit is instrumental in getting the circulation moving and helps when dealing with cellulite or varicose veins. For massage, combine 2 drops of grapefruit and 3 drops each of cypress and lemon in a tablespoon of carrier oil. Massage upward toward the heart.

When diffused, this sunny fruit oil relieves the ups and downs of PMS. Use it on its own or combine it in equal parts with cardamom and chamomile (Roman). For a headache, diffuse grapefruit in equal parts with peppermint and rosemary, or make a cool compress with these oils.

Personal Care and Well-Being

The astringent properties of grapefruit make it ideal for oily skin and hair. Use 6 or 7 drops in a quart of water for a facial steam that will open and cleanse the pores. After steaming, use a cotton ball to dab on a little astringent. Make the astringent with ¼ cup of cool chamomile tea, 1 tablespoon of witch hazel, and 5 drops each of grapefruit, carrot seed, and juniper berry. Grapefruit is also good for oily hair and promotes hair growth. Combine it with rosemary for an invigorating scalp massage.

Emotionally balancing, grapefruit is an aid for relieving nervous tension and exhaustion. Diffuse 3 parts grapefruit, 2 parts mandarin, and 1 part basil. This will also ease tension headaches,

· · · · · · · · ·

reduce irritability, and foster a sense of well-being. To help focus the mind, combine grapefruit with an equal amount of spearmint. This combination also helps you recover from jet lag or a hangover.

For support in meditation or spiritual practices, place a drop each of grapefruit, sandalwood, and lavender in the melted wax of a pillar or jar candle. For energy work, grapefruit activates the solar plexus and throat chakras. Use it in candle magic to attract abundance or for help in reaching goals.

For the Home

The antiseptic and antibacterial properties of grapefruit make it an ideal essential oil for cleaning kitchen surfaces. For extra power, combine it with lemongrass.

Grapefruit Kitchen Cleaner

2 cups water

2–4 tablespoons Castile soap

8 drops grapefruit essential oil

7 drops lemongrass essential oil

Combine all the ingredients in a spray bottle and gently shake to mix. To use, spray on surfaces and wipe off with a damp cloth.

Diffusing grapefruit removes stale odors. It is especially useful for keeping a refrigerator smelling clean and fresh. Combine 10 to 12 drops of it with an 8-ounce box of baking soda and mix well. For furniture and hardwood floors, add a few drops to a lemon cleaner. Test it on a small area first. For aromatic feng shui, use grapefruit to get energy moving.

ॐ Helichrysum ॐ

BOTANICAL NAME: *Helichrysum angustifolium* syn. *H. italicum*

ALSO KNOWN AS: Curry plant, everlasting, immortelle, Italian strawflower, whiteleaf

With branching stems that have been described as wand-like, helichrysum is a two-foot tall herb that is indigenous to the Mediterranean region. This shrubby plant has gray-green needle-like foliage and small yellow flowers that grow in domed clusters. The aroma of its leaves is reminiscent of curry. The flowers keep their fragrance and color even when dried, which is the source of the common names *everlasting* and *immortelle*. This has made helichrysum especially popular for dried flower arrangements and potpourri. The name *helichrysum* comes from the Greek and means "golden sun," in reference to the flowers that look like little round suns.[50]

From ancient times through the Middle Ages, helichrysum was used medicinally to treat a wide range of ailments. It was also used as a strewing herb to freshen homes. Today it is commonly used to scent cosmetics and soaps and as a fixative in perfumes.

Oil Description and Precautions

Steam distillation of the flower tops produces a pale yellow to reddish oil with a thin viscosity. It has an approximate shelf life of two to three years or slightly longer. This essential oil may cause skin irritation.

Blending for Scent

Helichrysum has a woody honey-like scent. It blends well with bergamot, black pepper, chamomile, clove bud, frankincense, lavender, mandarin, orange, palmarosa, rose, tea tree, and vetiver.

Scent Group	Perfume Note	Initial Strength	Sun Signs
Herbaceous	Middle to base	Strong	Gemini, Taurus

Medicinal Remedies

Helichrysum is used for acne, arthritis, asthma, boils, bronchitis, bruises, burns, bursitis, chapped skin, colds, coughs, cuts and scrapes, depression, dermatitis, eczema, fever, flu, inflammation, muscle aches and pains, poison ivy, rashes, scars, sprains and strains, stress, stretch marks, sunburn, and whooping cough.

The anti-inflammatory properties of helichrysum are effective to reduce the swelling and relieve the pain of sprains and strains. Combine 4 drops each of helichrysum and chamomile (German) in a tablespoon of carrier oil to gently massage the area. To release tight muscles and soothe joint pain, massage with 3 drops each of helichrysum and clary sage and 1 drop of clove bud in a tablespoon of carrier oil. For a massage mixture to relieve arthritis, use 1 drop each of helichrysum and fennel in a teaspoon of carrier oil.

Helichrysum's antiseptic properties make it ideal for first aid to disinfect cuts and scrapes. To treat a boil, make a warm compress with equal amounts of helichrysum and chamomile. Use helichrysum on its own for bruises or combine it with bay laurel. To soothe and heal a rash, use it in equal amounts with bergamot. In a steam inhalation, helichrysum helps to clear chest and nasal congestion and quiet coughs.

---

50. Coombes, *Dictionary of Plant Names*, 164.

Personal Care and Well-Being

When used in a facial moisturizer, helichrysum helps to tone and rejuvenate mature skin. It also helps oily skin, especially to reduce the inflammation of acne or the occasional pimple outbreak. Use 4 or 5 drops in a tablespoon of carrier oil for a cool compress to soothe puffy eyes. To relieve and heal sunburn, combine 2 tablespoons of aloe gel with 5 drops each of helichrysum and lavender. For dry, chapped hands, use 6 drops each of the same essential oils in 1 tablespoon each of coconut oil and shea butter.

Warming and grounding, the scent of helichrysum enhances well-being and helps dissolve emotional turmoil from the past. It brings a sense of peace as it balances energy, improving moods and mental clarity. In addition to balancing fluctuating moods, the following bath blend helps you overcome nervous exhaustion and deal with changes.

Helichrysum Mood-Boosting Bath Blend

2 cups Epsom or sea salt

2 tablespoons baking soda (optional)

4 tablespoons carrier oil or blend

5 drops helichrysum essential oil

5 drops bergamot essential oil

5 drops lavender essential oil

Place the dry ingredients in a glass or ceramic bowl. Combine the carrier and essential oils, add to the dry ingredients, and mix thoroughly.

For energy work, helichrysum activates the sacral, third eye, and crown chakras. The grounding effects of this oil help you prepare for meditation and prayer. It is effective for consecrating an altar or spiritual space. Use helichrysum in candle magic to attract prosperity. It also stimulates and enhances dreams.

For the Home

With antibacterial and antifungal properties, helichrysum will freshen and clean the air when diffused. It works well as a surface cleaner too. For aromatic feng shui, use helichrysum wherever you need to stimulate and move energy.

Hyssop

Botanical name: *Hyssopus officinalis*

Also known as: Hedge hyssop

Reaching approximately two feet in height, hyssop has upright angular stems. Its lance-shaped leaves are dark green, and its tiny purple-blue flowers grow in whorls at the ends of the stems. The stems, leaves, and flowers are aromatic. Native to the Mediterranean region, hyssop was highly regarded as a medicinal herb by the Greeks and Romans. Its genus and common names come from the Greek word *hussopos*, meaning "holy herb," referring to its use in cleaning temples.[51]

During the Middle Ages, priests used small branches of hyssop dipped in holy water to sprinkle blessings on their congregations. Hyssop also had mundane secular uses as a strewing herb for floors that were difficult to sweep and for stuffing mattresses. The common name *hedge hyssop* comes from its popularity as a clipped hedging plant in knot gardens.

Oil Description and Precautions

A colorless to pale yellow-green oil is produced by steam distillation of the leaves and flower tops. Hyssop has a thin viscosity and an approximate shelf life of two to three years. Avoid using this essential oil during pregnancy and while nursing; avoid if you have epilepsy or another seizure disorder; avoid with high blood pressure; may cause sensitization; use in moderation.

Blending for Scent

The scent of hyssop essential oil is slightly sweet and herbaceous, with camphoraceous undertones. It blends well with bay laurel, clary sage, geranium, lavender, lemon, lemon balm, lemongrass, lime, orange, and spearmint.

Scent Group	Perfume Note	Initial Strength	Sun Signs
Herbaceous	Middle to top	Medium	Cancer, Sagittarius

Medicinal Remedies

Hyssop is used for anxiety, arthritis, asthma, bronchitis, bruises, cold sores, colds, coughs, cuts and scrapes, dermatitis, eczema, flu, indigestion, inflammation, sore throat, stress, tonsillitis, and whooping cough.

The antiseptic and antiviral properties of hyssop are useful in treating cold sores. Combine 1 drop of hyssop in a teaspoon of carrier oil and apply with a cotton swab. Hyssop is effective

51. Kowalchik and Hylton, eds., *Rodale's Illustrated Encyclopedia of Herbs*, 342.

to relieve the inflammation of dermatitis and eczema. When used to clean cuts and wounds, it helps reduce scarring. To treat bruises, combine a tablespoon of carrier oil with 3 drops each of hyssop and palmarosa and 2 drops of clove bud. Combining it with lavender also works well to reduce bruising.

Hyssop is especially good for treating the chest and nasal congestion of colds and flu. Diffuse it with peppermint, rosemary, and thyme to bring relief and clean the air. The same combination of essential oils also makes an effective chest rub.

Congestion-Clearing Hyssop Diffuser Blend

2 parts hyssop essential oil

2 parts peppermint essential oil

1 part rosemary essential oil

1 part thyme essential oil

Combine the oils, then place in the diffuser.

The antispasmodic and expectorant properties of hyssop can help relieve bronchial spasms. Make a steam inhalation with 3 drops each of hyssop, spearmint, and cajeput in a quart of water. For a sore throat, use 4 drops each of hyssop and geranium in a steam inhalation. For cold relief on the go, use 4 drops each of hyssop and thyme in an inhaler.

Personal Care and Well-Being

Hyssop is an aid for relaxation, helping to release anxiety, nervous tension, and stress. For an uplifting combination, diffuse it in equal parts with lavender and lemon balm to melt away tension. For a relaxing massage to alleviate mental fatigue, combine 5 drops of lavender with 4 drops each of hyssop and juniper berry in an ounce of carrier oil. To clear the mind and bring clarity to emotions, diffuse 2 parts each of hyssop and lemon with 1 part ylang-ylang.

For energy work, hyssop activates the sacral, solar plexus, and throat chakras.

Because of its long history of use in cleaning sacred spaces, hyssop is ideal for purifying and preparing an altar or sacred space. It also lends support for meditation and spiritual practices. Use hyssop in candle magic to remove any form of negativity.

For the Home

In addition to working as a general insect repellent, hyssop is especially effective for deterring flies when diffused. To discourage moths in a closet or storage container, make a sachet with ½ cup of baking soda and 15 drops of hyssop. For aromatic feng shui, use hyssop to stimulate energy.

• • • • • • •

✌ Juniper Berry ⌇

BOTANICAL NAME: *Juniperus communis*

ALSO KNOWN AS: Common juniper, gin berry

Frequently used in landscaping, juniper is an evergreen shrub with spreading branches that grows up to six feet tall. Young junipers have needle-like leaves, while mature ones usually have scale-like foliage. The round juniper berry is technically a cone. Taking about two years to mature, berries turn from green to blue-black and frequently have a light dusting of white powder.

In addition to using juniper berries medicinally, the Romans flavored their food with them when black pepper was unavailable. In medieval Europe, juniper boughs were burned to fumigate homes for protection against the plague and other diseases. This practice continued up until World War I, when juniper was burned to help fight epidemics. Juniper berries are well known for their use as flavoring in stews and roasts. They also provide the distinctive taste of gin. The scent of juniper is widely used in perfumes, soaps, and cosmetics.

Oil Description and Precautions

Steam distillation of unripe juniper berries produces a white or pale yellow oil. It has a thin viscosity and an approximate shelf life of two to three years. Avoid using this essential oil during pregnancy; avoid with kidney disease; may cause slight skin irritation; use in moderation.

Blending for Scent

Juniper berry has a sweetly woody and balsamic scent. It blends well with bergamot, black pepper, clary sage, cypress, elemi, fir needle, geranium, lavender, lemongrass, pine, rosemary, sandalwood, and vetiver.

Scent Group	Perfume Note	Initial Strength	Sun Signs
Woody	Middle	Medium	Aries, Leo, Sagittarius

Medicinal Remedies

Juniper berry is used for acne, anxiety, arthritis, bursitis, cellulite, colds, cuts and scrapes, dermatitis, eczema, flu, gout, hangover, hemorrhoids, muscle aches and pains, psoriasis, and stress.

To reduce cellulite, massage with 2 drops each of juniper berry, cypress, and grapefruit in a tablespoon of carrier oil. To ease the discomfort of gout, use juniper berry, basil, and carrot seed for a massage blend. For arthritis, combine juniper berry with ginger and clove bud.

Juniper Bursitis-Busting Gel

2 tablespoons aloe gel

6 drops juniper essential oil

2 drops cypress essential oil

2 drops marjoram essential oil

Mix ingredients thoroughly. Store in a jar with a tight-fitting lid.

The combination of essential oils that ease bursitis also works well in a warm compress for joints affected by arthritis. Use 3 drops of cypress and 1 drop each of juniper berry and marjoram in a tablespoon of carrier oil in a quart of hot water. For muscles that ache after exertion, use juniper berry on its own to make a warm compress.

To soothe and heal skin conditions such as dermatitis, eczema, or psoriasis, make a bath oil with 5 drops each of juniper berry, chamomile, and carrot seed in an ounce of carrier oil. For psoriasis of the scalp, use 1 drop each of the same essential oils in a tablespoon of carrier oil and gently massage into the scalp. Leave it on for about ten minutes, then shampoo and rinse well.

Following the age-old practice of using juniper to fumigate against illness, diffuse it in equal amounts with eucalyptus (blue) and lemon to clean the air of a sickroom. This will also help relieve the respiratory discomfort of colds.

Personal Care and Well-Being

The astringent properties of juniper make it ideal for oily skin, helping to unblock pores and balance oils. Make a skin toner with ¼ cup of cool chamomile tea and 6 drops each of juniper and rosemary. Pour into a bottle with a cap and shake well. Apply it to your face with a cotton ball. Juniper berry is also helpful for oily hair.

This essential oil is effective in calming nervous tension and recovering from exhaustion. Diffuse 2 parts juniper berry and 1 part each of bergamot and ginger to revitalize emotions and lift moods. The crisp scent of juniper supports a general sense of well-being. In energy work, it activates the sacral, solar plexus, and third eye chakras.

This oil helps to ground and center energy for meditation and prayer and enhances spiritual practices. In candle magic, use juniper berry to attract abundance and happiness. It also removes negativity and fosters success. In addition to supporting restful sleep, it enhances dream work.

For the Home

Juniper works well as a room spray or carpet powder to freshen and remove stale odors. It also is an insect repellent. Add a few drops to a citronella candle to add power and aroma. Use juniper berry for aromatic feng shui wherever you need to get energy moving.

• • • • • • •

❧ Lavender ❧

BOTANICAL NAME: *Lavandula angustifolia*, syn. *L. officinalis*
ALSO KNOWN AS: Common lavender, English lavender, garden lavender, true lavender

Lavender is a bushy evergreen shrub that reaches two to three feet in height and spreads about two feet wide. Small purplish-lavender flowers grow in whorls atop leafless spikes. The slightly fuzzy leaves are narrow and gray or silvery green. Lavender has been a well-known and loved fragrance since ancient times. The Greeks and Romans used it for treating a range of ailments and for cleaning their homes. The Romans introduced the plant into England, where it became a mainstay of gardens.

Throughout Europe during the Middles Ages, lavender was popular for medicinal purposes and as a strewing herb to freshen homes, especially sickrooms. Sachets of lavender were used to scent linens and deter moths, fleas, and other pests. Soap maker William of Yardley knew a good thing when he saw it (or smelled it) and managed to get a monopoly on England's lavender. Not willing to part with this beloved garden plant, the Pilgrims brought it with them to North America.

Oil Description and Precautions

Produced by steam distillation of the flower tops, lavender essential oil ranges from colorless to pale yellow. It has a thin viscosity and an approximate shelf life of two to three years or slightly longer. Do not use lavender essential oil when taking sedative medications.

There are several types of lavender, which makes it important to purchase the right one for the purposes described here. Spanish lavender (*L. stoechas*) is stimulating and has the opposite effect of English lavender. In addition, it is sometimes marketed under the same botanical name as English lavender but called *French lavender*.

Blending for Scent

Lavender essential oil has a herbaceous floral scent with balsamic woody undertones. It goes well with so many oils, but some that it blends particularly well with include bay laurel, black pepper, cajeput, cedarwood, citrus (any type), cypress, elemi, fir needle, geranium, juniper berry, marjoram, palmarosa, patchouli, peppermint, pine, rosemary, and vetiver.

Scent Group	Perfume Note	Initial Strength	Sun Signs
Floral	Middle to top	Strong	Aquarius, Gemini, Leo, Pisces, Virgo

Medicinal Remedies

Lavender is used for acne, anxiety, arthritis, asthma, athlete's foot, blisters, boils, bronchitis, bruises, burns, chapped skin, chilblains, colds, coughs, cuts and scrapes, depression, dermatitis, earache, eczema, flu, head lice, headaches, indigestion, inflammation, insect bites and stings, insomnia, laryngitis, menopausal discomforts, menstrual cramps, migraines, muscle aches and pains, nausea, poison ivy, premenstrual syndrome (PMS), psoriasis, rashes, ringworm, scabies, scars, sore throat, sprains and strains, stress, stretch marks, sunburn, vertigo, and whooping cough.

As previously mentioned, French chemist René-Maurice Gattefossé rediscovered the healing power of lavender essential oil after burning his hand in the laboratory. As a nod to his discovery, make a salve to keep on hand as first aid for burns. Lavender is a skin rejuvenator that relieves pain and heals without scarring. The salve can also be used for cuts and to soothe the inflammation of skin disorders such as psoriasis, eczema, and dermatitis. It is also effective for healing boils and bruises.

Lavender Burn Ointment

½ ounce beeswax, grated or shaved

6 tablespoons carrier oil or blend

1 teaspoon lavender essential oil

Place the beeswax and carrier oil in a jar in a saucepan of water. Warm it over low heat, stirring until the wax melts. Remove it from the heat and allow the mixture to cool to room temperature before adding the essential oil. Adjust the consistency if necessary. Let the mixture cool completely before using or storing.

To soothe poison ivy, mix 2 drops of lavender with 1 drop of frankincense in a teaspoon of carrier oil. For bee stings, combine lavender with eucalyptus (blue).

Not only is lavender relaxing for massage, but its analgesic properties make it especially effective to relieve muscle pain and stiff joints. For healing bath salts, combine 10 drops of lavender with 3 drops each of chamomile (German) and coriander in 4 tablespoons of carrier oil. Mix thoroughly with 2 cups of Epsom salt. For sprains and strains, make a compress with 3 drops each of lavender and rosemary in a tablespoon of carrier oil and add it to a quart of water. To combat nausea, use 5 drops each of lavender and peppermint in an inhaler.

Personal Care and Well-Being

Lavender soap is popular not only because of its scent but also because it is especially good for the skin. Lavender is appropriate to use on any skin type. Its antiseptic properties make it ideal for a cleansing facial steam to deal with pimple outbreaks. Lavender helps balance scalp oils and control dandruff. Combine it with rosemary to soothe the itching of dandruff. It aids in hair growth and is appropriate to use on normal hair. With antibacterial properties, it works well in a deodorant too.

Lavender may be best known for balancing emotions and fostering a sense of peaceful calm, especially when dealing with grief. For energy work, use it to activate any individual chakra or balance all of them. Lavender supports meditation and prayer. When used in candle magic, it can foster and enhance love.

For the Home

Used for laundering since Roman times, lavender not only freshens clothes and linens but also helps clean and deodorize the washing machine. It deters moths in the linen closet, keeps mosquitoes away outdoors, and disrupts ant trails in the home. For aromatic feng shui, use it to calm and balance energy.

❧ Lemon ❧

BOTANICAL NAME: *Citrus limon* syn. *C. limonum*

Indigenous to India, China, and Myanmar, the lemon tree was valued for medicinal purposes and treasured for its fragrance in ancient times. Originally cultivated in the Indus Valley, it was grown in Iran between 2500 and 500 BCE and then in Greece.[52] During the Middle Ages, lemon trees were grown as much for their beauty as for practical use of the fruit. Used throughout Europe for a wide range of complaints, lemons were considered a potent cure-all and became standard cargo on British naval ships, especially for preventing scurvy.

Reaching only about twenty feet tall, the lemon tree has sharp thorns growing along its twigs. Its leaves are dark green on top and light green underneath. Starting as mildly fragrant reddish buds, the white flowers remain tinged with pink. The French word *citron*, "lemon," came from Latin and was a name applied to all citrus fruits and trees. The Greek word *kitrion* is thought to have been derived from *kedris*, "cedar cone," referring to the appearance of the immature fruit.[53]

Oil Description and Precautions

Cold-pressing the entire fruit produces a pale greenish-yellow oil with a thin viscosity. It has an approximate shelf life of nine to twelve months. This essential oil may cause skin irritation or sensitization; it is phototoxic.

---

52. Cumo, ed., *Encyclopedia of Cultivated Plants*, 564.
53. Sonneman, *Lemon: A Global History*, 13.

Blending for Scent

Lemon essential oil has a lightly fruity and citrus scent. It blends especially well with cardamom, chamomile, eucalyptus, fennel, geranium, juniper berry, neroli, rose, and sandalwood.

Scent Group	Perfume Note	Initial Strength	Sun Signs
Citrus	Top	Very strong	Aquarius, Cancer, Gemini, Pisces

Medicinal Remedies

Lemon essential oil is used for acne, arthritis, asthma, blisters, boils, bronchitis, cellulite, chilblains, circulation, cold sores, colds, corns and calluses, coughs, cuts and scrapes, fever, flu, gout, hangover, headaches, insect bites and stings, jet lag, varicose veins, and warts.

With a wide range of uses, lemon is a good essential oil to keep on hand. To ease the chest congestion of colds and coughs, make a steam inhalation with 4 drops of lemon, 2 drops of eucalyptus (blue), and 1 drop of cypress. Lemon's antiseptic and antibacterial properties make it ideal as a styptic for minor cuts.

To ease cold sores, mix 3 drops of lemon and 2 drops of manuka in a tablespoon of carrier oil. To relieve a headache, diffuse equal amounts of lemon, lavender, and peppermint. To alleviate jet lag or a hangover, use lemon in equal amounts with ginger.

Personal Care and Well-Being

Lemon's astringent and antibacterial properties are ideal for oily skin, especially during pimple outbreaks. For a deep-cleaning facial steam, use it in equal amounts with lavender.

In addition to treating dandruff, lemon stimulates the scalp and balances oils. It also adds shine and is appropriate for normal hair too. Mix 4 drops in a tablespoon of carrier oil, massage into the scalp, then shampoo and rinse well. Because it fights bacteria, lemon makes a good ingredient for deodorant.

Lemon fosters a sense of well-being. Diffuse it in equal amounts with rosemary when you need help concentrating, or add a little peppermint for a trio of oils to lift moods. Combine lemon with bergamot and anise seed for clear thinking. When dealing with exhaustion, mix lemon with basil and mandarin.

For energy work, lemon stimulates the solar plexus, heart, and third eye chakras. It provides general support for meditation and spiritual practices. Use lemon in candle magic to attract prosperity, foster happiness, and gain success.

For the Home

Lemon is a heavyweight when it comes to cleaning. It makes an excellent window cleaner when combined with vinegar and water. For a powerful surface cleaner, combine it with rosemary and tea tree. On its own or in equal amounts with lavender, lemon helps to clean and freshen a washing machine.

Lemon Washing Machine Wash

3–4 cups white vinegar

½ cup baking soda

30 drops lemon essential oil

Set the washer to large load with hot water. Let it fill, add all the ingredients, and allow the machine to agitate for a minute. Stop the wash cycle and let it sit for about forty-five minutes. Next, dip a cloth in the water and wipe around the top of the tub and the bleach and fabric softener dispensers. Then allow the wash and rinse cycles to finish.

Combine 20 drops of lemon with 2 ounces of beeswax to make a furniture polish. Apply it to a small area to test. Add a few drops of lemon to a citronella candle for extra scent and to help keep mosquitoes away. For feng shui, use lemon wherever you need to stimulate energy.

❧ Lemon Balm ❧

BOTANICAL NAME: *Melissa officinalis*

ALSO KNOWN AS: Bee balm, common balm, honey plant, Melissa, mint balm, sweet balm

Reaching up to three feet tall, this bushy herb has bright green leaves with a noticeable lemony scent. Small white to yellowish flowers grow in clusters along the stems. Known widely as *Melissa*, Greek for "bee," lemon balm attracts and calms them, which is why beekeepers have grown it near their hives for over two thousand years.[54]

An important medicinal herb during the Middle Ages, lemon balm was used for a wide range of ailments. Even though herbalists Culpeper and Gerard touted its power, lemon balm's popularity was not carried to the New World. Its rediscovery had to wait for the resurgence of herbal medicine during the late twentieth century. Lemon balm is widely used in commercial skin care products.

Oil Description and Precautions

Ranging from pale to full yellow, lemon balm essential oil is produced by steam distillation of the leaves and flower tops. It has a thin viscosity and an approximate shelf life of two to three years. This essential oil may cause skin irritation or sensitization.

---

54. Castleman, *The New Healing Herbs*, 305.

Blending for Scent

As expected, lemon balm's scent is lemony but also fresh and herbaceous. Some oils that blend well with it include chamomile, frankincense, geranium, lavender, neroli, peppermint, petitgrain, rose, and spearmint.

Scent Group	Perfume Note	Initial Strength	Sun Sign
Citrus	Middle	Strong	Cancer

Medicinal Remedies

Lemon balm is used for anxiety, asthma, bronchitis, coughs, depression, eczema, fever, hay fever, headaches, indigestion, inflammation, insect bites and stings, insomnia, menstrual cramps, migraines, nausea, premenstrual syndrome (PMS), seasonal affective disorder (SAD), stress, and sunburn.

To help ease coughs, including bronchitis, combine lemon balm and peppermint in equal amounts for a steam inhalation to help clear the airways. For a chest rub, combine 3 drops each of lemon balm and ginger and 2 drops of eucalyptus (blue) in a tablespoon of jojoba.

Take the inflammation and itchy discomfort out of eczema by mixing 1 drop of lemon balm in a teaspoon of carrier oil and applying it to the affected area. This remedy can also be used to relieve the swelling and itching of insect bites and stings. It is especially effective on wasp stings. For extra power, blend lemon balm with lavender and bergamot to keep on hand.

Soothing Lemon Balm Oil

2 drops bergamot essential oil

5 drops lemon balm essential oil

5 drops lavender essential oil

2 tablespoons apricot kernel carrier oil

Mix the essential oils together and combine with the carrier oil. Store any leftover oil in a bottle with a tight-fitting cap.

As an alternative for dealing with eczema, use lemon balm with sea or Epsom salt for a healing soak in the tub. For a calming soak before bed, combine lemon balm and clary sage to relax and aid in getting a good night's sleep.

Diffusing lemon balm is effective to reduce anxiety and relieve headaches. For aid in relieving PMS symptoms, use it in equal amounts with cardamom or coriander. For seasonal affective disorder, diffuse 2 parts lemon balm and 1 part each of orange and ylang-ylang.

Personal Care and Well-Being

Lemon balm can be used for all skin types. Its antioxidants aid mature complexions, and its anti-bacterial properties help oily skin and the occasional pimple outbreak. With extra dilution, it can be used on sensitive skin. It is a good skin toner: combine 15 drops of lemon balm in ¼ cup of chamomile tea in a bottle, then shake well and apply with a cotton ball.

Lemon balm helps calm the nerves and is especially helpful when coping with sudden changes in life. Combine 4 drops of lemon balm, 3 drops of vetiver, and 2 drops of chamomile (Roman) in a tablespoon of carrier oil to massage on your temples. Lemon balm on its own aids concentration and mental clarity. When dealing with grief, diffuse 2 parts each of lemon balm and orange and 1 part frankincense. This combination of oils also fosters a sense of peace.

When engaging in energy work, lemon balm stimulates the sacral and heart chakras. Also use it for general support of meditation and spiritual practices. For candle magic, lemon balm helps to foster happiness, attract love, and attain success. It is also supportive for dream and past-life work.

For the Home

To deter insects from entering your home, make lemon balm candles or use it in a reed diffuser near an open window. On the patio, add a few drops to a citronella candle to enhance the scent and add to its effectiveness. For feng shui, use lemon balm salts or candles to maintain balance after calming or stimulating the energy.

The Lemongrass Oils

Lemongrass is a tropical aromatic grass with a pungent, lemony fragrance. With long, narrow leaf blades, it grows in large, dense clumps that can reach up to five feet tall and four feet wide. Inconspicuous greenish flowers grow atop narrow stalks. The genus name, *Cymbopogon*, comes from the Greek words *kymbe* and *pogon*, meaning "boat" and "beard," respectively, and refers to the flowers and bracts (modified leaves) that enclose the flowers.[55]

Both types of lemongrass, East Indian and West Indian, have been cultivated for centuries as culinary and medicinal herbs. Lemongrass has a long history of use in India for treating fever and infectious diseases and to freshen homes. The following lemongrass essential oils are used interchangeably for therapeutic purposes.

---

55. Foster and Johnson, *National Geographic Desk Reference to Nature's Medicine*, 228.

✍ Lemongrass, East Indian ✍

BOTANICAL NAME: *Cymbopogon flexuosus*

ALSO KNOWN AS: British Indian lemongrass, fever tea, French Indian verbena

Native to eastern India, this lemongrass is now cultivated in the western part of the country, where it is called *fever tea*. Its species name means "winding," referring to the way its roots grow in a zigzag pattern.[56]

Oil Description and Precautions

A yellow or amber oil is produced by steam distillation of the leaves. It has a thin viscosity and an approximate shelf life of twelve to eighteen months. This essential oil may cause skin irritation; do not use around the eyes; do not use on babies or children under six years old; avoid during pregnancy.

Blending for Scents

This lemongrass has a grassy, lemony scent that is lighter than that of its West Indian cousin. It blends well with basil, black pepper, cedarwood, fennel, geranium, lavender, marjoram, orange, palmarosa, rosemary, and vetiver.

Scent Group	Perfume Note	Initial Strength	Sun Sign
Citrus	Middle to top	Very strong	Gemini

✍ Lemongrass, West Indian ✍

BOTANICAL NAME: *Cymbopogon citratus* syn. *Andropogon citratus*

ALSO KNOWN AS: Citronella grass, Madagascar lemongrass, West Indian lemongrass

Native to Sri Lanka, this lemongrass is now cultivated in the West Indies, Africa, and tropical Asia. As its species name implies, it has a very citrus-like scent, which may be familiar to many of us who grew up using Ivory soap.

Oil Description and Precautions

The leaves are steam-distilled, producing an oil that can be yellow, amber, or reddish brown. It has a thin viscosity and an approximate shelf life of twelve to eighteen months. This essential oil

---

56. Neal, *Gardener's Latin*, 53.

may cause skin irritation; do not use around the eyes; do not use on babies or children under six years old; avoid during pregnancy.

Blending for Scent

This lemongrass has a fresh citrus and grassy scent with earthy undertones. It blends well with basil, bergamot, cedarwood, coriander, geranium, lavender, marjoram, orange, tea tree, and thyme.

Scent Group	Perfume Note	Initial Strength	Sun Sign
Citrus	Middle to top	Very strong	Gemini

Medicinal Remedies for Both Lemongrass Oils

The lemongrass oils are used for acne, athlete's foot, circulation, colds, fever, flu, head lice, headaches, indigestion, insect bites and stings, jet lag, jock itch, muscle aches and pain, scabies, sprains and strains, stress, tendinitis, vaginal infection, and varicose veins.

Lemongrass contains many of the same insect-repellent compounds as its relative citronella (*C. nardus*) and has been used to repel fleas, ticks, and lice. In advance of an outing, make a spray that you can apply at home and take with you. Combine 4 drops of lemongrass and ½ teaspoon of carrier oil in a spray bottle with 2 ounces of water. Shake well before each use.

If you didn't make a spray before heading outside, combine lemongrass with spearmint to soothe insect bites and stings when you get home. Lemongrass can also be used in the bath to treat scabies.

The analgesic properties of lemongrass help to ease general muscle pain, sprains and strains, and tendinitis. Combine it with vetiver and rosemary to boost its effectiveness.

Lemongrass Pain Reliever Blend

4 drops lemongrass essential oil

3 drops rosemary essential oil

2 drops vetiver essential oil

2 tablespoons carrier oil or blend

Mix the essential oils and combine with the carrier oil. Store any leftover oil in a bottle with a tight-fitting cap.

Personal Care and Well-Being

Lemongrass works well to brighten and tone the complexion. Its antiseptic and astringent properties are good for normal, oily, and acne-prone skin. Combine it with geranium and lavender to deal with flare-ups. Lemongrass helps to balance scalp oils, too. With its antibacterial properties,

· · · · · · · ·

it is ideal as an ingredient in deodorant. When used in the bath, it helps with excessive perspiration by opening the pores and fighting bacteria.

To relieve headaches, mental fatigue, nervous exhaustion, or stress, use lemongrass on its own or diffuse it in equal amounts with lavender and chamomile. To refresh the mind and gain clarity, diffuse 2 parts each of lemongrass and orange with 1 part basil. For energy work, lemongrass activates the root, solar plexus, and throat chakras. It is useful for grounding and centering before meditation and prayer. In candle magic, use lemongrass to attract luck.

For the Home

Use lemongrass for feng shui to stimulate energy in your home. To scent the air and keep insects out of the house or away from a patio area while dining, combine equal amounts of lemongrass, lavender, and peppermint. A festive way to use the oils is to make scented ribbons. Cut foot-long strips of cotton ribbons, dip them in the essential oil blend (there is no need to use a carrier oil for this), then hang them in open windows or around your patio. If ribbons aren't your thing, use the blend in a diffuser or candles.

❧ Lime ❧

BOTANICAL NAME: *Citrus aurantifolia*

ALSO KNOWN AS: Key lime, Mexican lime, sour lime, West Indian lime

The lime from which essential oil is extracted is not the same as those found in most supermarkets, which are Persian limes (*C. latifolia*). The key lime is believed to have originated in India or the Malay Archipelago. It was transported to the Middle East by Arab merchants, into Europe by returning Crusaders, and then to the Caribbean in the sixteenth century by the Spanish. Becoming popular in North America in the early 1900s, this lime was named for the Florida Keys, where it was grown.[57] After being mostly wiped out by a hurricane, the Persian lime became the replacement crop.

Since the tenth century, lime has been used medicinally for a range of issues and to prevent scurvy. Discovering that limes worked as well as lemons, the British Navy dispensed lime with rum rations and earned their sailors the nickname "Limey."

Although the botanical name is frequently written with a multiplication sign (*Citrus × aurantiifolia*), there is no hard proof that this tree is a hybrid. Its species name means "leaves like the orange."[58] Key lime is a small evergreen tree with sharp spines. It has oval leaves and white flowers.

---

57. Cumo, ed., *Encyclopedia of Cultivated Plants*, 592.
58. Coombes, *Dictionary of Plant Names*, 56.

• • • • • • •

Oil Description and Precautions

Two essential oils are obtained from limes: one from the peel and one from the whole fruit. Cold-pressing the peel produces a pale yellow to olive-green oil with a thin viscosity and an approximate shelf life of nine to twelve months. Oil extracted from only the peel is phototoxic.

Steam-distilling the whole ripe fruit produces a white to pale yellow oil. It also has a thin viscosity and an approximate shelf life of nine to twelve months.

Blending for Scent

Essential oil from the peel has a sweet citrus scent; oil from the whole fruit smells fruity and clean. Some scents that both lime oils blend well with include black pepper, citronella, clary sage, elemi, ginger, lavender, neroli, peppermint, rosemary, and ylang-ylang.

Scent Group	Perfume Note	Initial Strength	Sun Sign
Citrus	Top	Medium	Leo

Medicinal Remedies

Lime essential oil is used for acne, arthritis, asthma, boils, bronchitis, cellulite, chilblains, circulation, cold sores, colds, corns and calluses, coughs, cuts and scrapes, fever, flu, insect bites and stings, varicose veins, and warts.

Lime's antibacterial and antiviral properties make it effective in treating respiratory ailments. When used in a steam inhalation, it eases coughs and colds while helping to open the sinus and bronchial airways. Swish 6 drops of the oil into a quart of steaming water. Alternatively, combine it with peppermint (3 drops each) for powerful relief. To help bring down a fever, make a compress with 6 or 7 drops of lime in a quart of cool water.

In addition to colds and flu, cold weather brings the potential for chilblains, which are itchy swellings that develop on the skin in response to cold temperatures. The gentle application of a selection of oils can relieve the pain and itching and heal the skin.

Lime Chilblain Relief

1 tablespoon carrier oil or blend

3 drops lime essential oil

2 drops chamomile essential oil

2 drops lavender essential oil

1 drop black pepper essential oil

Combine all the oils and mix well. Store any leftover oil in a bottle with a tight-fitting cap.

• • • • • • • •

Lime is also an aid when dealing with the pain and swelling of varicose veins. Use 8 drops of lime and 6 drops of cypress in an ounce of carrier oil for a soothing soak in the tub. To relieve gout or arthritis, make a massage oil with 4 drops of lime and 2 drops each of juniper berry and rosemary in a tablespoon of carrier oil.

Personal Care and Well-Being

Lime balances oily skin and brightens a dull complexion. Its antiseptic and astringent properties help to clear pimple outbreaks. For the hair, add 1 or 2 drops to your shampoo to help balance scalp oils and add shine. For a scalp massage to treat dandruff, combine 4 drops of lime, 2 drops of lavender, and 1 drop of mandarin with 2 tablespoons of carrier oil.

The uplifting scent of lime is an aid for bringing emotions into balance and fostering a sense of well-being. For an energizing diffuser blend to lift mental fatigue, combine 3 parts lime, 2 parts bergamot, and 1 part rosemary. For energy work, use lime to activate the heart and throat chakras. It is also effective when preparing for meditation or prayer. In candle magic, lime attracts love, fosters abundance, and aids in reaching goals.

For the Home

Because it kills bacteria, lime not only deodorizes a room when used in a diffuser but also cleans the air. Its crisp citrusy scent is especially nice during the winter months. Lime also makes a good kitchen and bath surface cleaner. Add 15 drops of it to 1 cup of water and 1 cup of white vinegar. For aromatic feng shui, use lime to get energy moving.

✺ Mandarin ✺

BOTANICAL NAME: *Citrus reticulata* syn. *C. nobilis*

ALSO KNOWN AS: European mandarin, mandarin orange, true mandarin

Although they were first planted in Europe during the early 1800s, mandarins have been cultivated in China for over four thousand years.[59] The fruit was possibly named for the civil servants called *mandarins* who wore yellow robes. The species name comes from the Latin *reticulate*, meaning "netted," which refers to the white net-patterned pith underneath the peel.[60] This small spiny tree has slender branches and glossy oval leaves. Its white flowers are very fragrant.

The terms *mandarin* and *tangerine* are often used interchangeably because the fruit are nearly indistinguishable to the layperson, plus they share the same botanical name. However, mandarin is the name given to a class of oranges that are easy to peel. Tangerine is regarded as a subgroup of mandarin or a type of mandarin with darker reddish-orange skin.

---

59. Khan, ed., *Citrus Genetics, Breeding and Biotechnology*, 26.

60. Neal, *Gardener's Latin*, 105.

Oil Description and Precautions

The peel is cold-pressed, producing a greenish-orange oil with a thin viscosity. It has an approximate shelf life of nine to twelve months. While mandarin essential oil is generally regarded as safe, it may be phototoxic for people with sensitive skin.

Blending for Scent

Mandarin essential oil has a sweet, fruity, and almost floral scent. Some oils that blend well with it include anise seed, bergamot, clary sage, clove bud, elemi, frankincense, lavender, neroli, and ylang-ylang.

Scent Group	Perfume Note	Initial Strength	Sun Sign
Citrus	Top	Medium	Aquarius

Medicinal Remedies

Mandarin is used for acne, constipation, hangover, indigestion, insomnia, nausea, scars, stress, and stretch marks.

To combat nausea, especially morning sickness, place 10 drops of mandarin and 5 drops of peppermint in an inhaler to take with you. This combination is also helpful for clearing the cobwebs of a hangover. To diminish the appearance of scars and stretch marks, combine 3 drops each of mandarin, helichrysum, and lavender with a tablespoon of rosehip seed carrier oil. For dealing with stress, diffuse 2 parts mandarin and 1 part cardamom. For insomnia, diffuse it with sandalwood.

Personal Care and Well-Being

Mandarin works well as a toner for mature skin and helps combat wrinkles. Combine ¼ cup of cool herb tea, 8 drops of mandarin, and 3 drops each of frankincense and lavender. Shake well and apply with a cotton ball. Mandarin's astringent properties are an aid for oily skin and the occasional pimple outbreak. For help dealing with dandruff, add 4 drops of mandarin to a tablespoon of carrier oil to massage into the scalp.

While mandarin is not used for a wide range of physical ailments, it is a powerhouse when it comes to the mind and emotions. When dealing with mental fatigue and nervous tension, diffuse 3 parts mandarin and 2 parts each of cedarwood and palmarosa. To foster a sense of well-being, use 3 parts mandarin, 2 parts lavender, and 1 part ginger. Of course, there's nothing like a soak in the tub to quiet emotional turmoil and lift your spirits, especially if you use a couple of fizzy bath bombs.

Uplifting Mandarin Bath Bombs

1 cup baking soda

½ cup citric acid

1 teaspoon dried herbs and/or flower petals (optional)

½ teaspoon cocoa butter

6 drops mandarin essential oil

2 drops frankincense essential oil

2 drops ylang-ylang essential oil

1–2 drops carrier oil (if necessary)

Combine the dry ingredients and set aside. Boil a little water in a saucepan and remove it from the heat. Place the cocoa butter in a jar in the water and stir until melted. Allow it to cool, then stir in the essential oils. Slowly mix in the dry ingredients until the mixture has the consistency of clumpy wet sand. Add a drop or two of carrier oil if the mixture is too dry. Press it into decorative candy molds and let sit for a day. A melon baller can also be used to shape the bath bombs. Let the balls sit on a piece of wax paper for a day. Store them in a jar with a tight-fitting lid.

When working with the chakras, use mandarin to activate the solar plexus, heart, and throat energy centers. Mandarin provides gentle support for meditation and spiritual practices. For candle magic, use it to attract abundance, foster happiness, or reach a goal.

For the Home

For a delightful air freshener, diffuse 3 parts mandarin and 2 parts each of chamomile and geranium. Mandarin works nicely in a linen closet sachet on its own or in equal amounts with lavender. Mix 15 drops of each oil with a cup of baking soda. For aromatic feng shui, use mandarin wherever you need to calm fast-moving energy.

✄ Manuka ✄

BOTANICAL NAME: *Leptospermum scoparium*

ALSO KNOWN AS: Broom tree, New Zealand tea tree, tea bush

Native to New Zealand and Australia, the manuka is a shrubby evergreen tree with silver-gray needle-like leaves. Growing along the branches among the leaves, the flowers range from white to reddish and have dark red centers. Its botanical name comes from the Greek words *leptos*, meaning "slender," and *sperma*, "seed," referring to the narrow seeds, and the Latin word *scoparium*, "broom-like." [61]

For centuries, the Maori used the leaves for medicinal purposes as well as for a refreshment tea. British explorer Captain James Cook (1728–1779) hoped manuka would help alleviate scurvy and took samples back to England. On his second voyage to New Zealand, his crew was more creative and used the leaves to brew beer.

Oil Description and Precautions

The leaves and twigs are steam-distilled, producing an oil that ranges from clear to amber. It has a medium viscosity and a slightly oily texture. Manuka has an approximate shelf life of two to three years. This essential oil is generally regarded as safe.

Blending for Scent

Manuka has a herbaceous, woodsy scent with a sweet honey-like undertone. Some oils that blend well with it include basil, chamomile, cypress, eucalyptus, geranium, grapefruit, lavender, lemon, mandarin, peppermint, petitgrain, pine, sandalwood, and tea tree.

Scent Group	Perfume Note	Initial Strength	Sun Signs
Herbaceous	Middle	Medium	Capricorn, Pisces, Sagittarius

Medicinal Remedies

Manuka is used for acne, anxiety, athlete's foot, chicken pox, cold sores, colds, coughs, cuts and scrapes, flu, hay fever, headaches, insect bites and stings, jock itch, migraines, muscle aches and pains, ringworm, sinus infection, stress, vaginal infection, warts, and whooping cough.

Like other essential oils from "down under," manuka helps relieve the chest and nasal congestion of colds. Use it on its own for a steam inhalation, or combine 4 drops each of manuka and eucalyptus (lemon) in a quart of water. Manuka is an expectorant that helps clear respiratory airways.

To massage away the muscle aches related to cold and flu, mix 4 drops each of manuka and eucalyptus (blue) in a tablespoon of carrier oil. For relief from hay fever, use manuka in equal parts with chamomile and lemon balm in a diffuser or an inhaler.

With antibacterial and antiseptic properties, manuka is a good choice for a first aid ointment to fight infection. Use it in equal amounts with lavender to enhance the scent and the healing power. When bitten or stung by insects, mix 3 drops of manuka in a teaspoon of carrier oil to apply to the site. It is especially effective for treating spider and tick bites.

---

61. Coombes, *Dictionary of Plant Names*, 116.

· · · · · · · ·

Personal Care and Well-Being

Perfect for oily skin, manuka's antibacterial and anti-inflammatory properties are particularly helpful for pimple outbreaks. Make a facial scrub with a teaspoon of finely ground oatmeal, 2 to 3 drops of carrier oil, and 1 or 2 drops of manuka. Gently massage it on your face, then rinse with lukewarm water. Manuka soothes itchy dandruff and helps fight foot and body odor when used in the bath.

Manuka helps control anger and stabilize emotional turmoil. Diffuse it with 3 parts chamomile and 2 parts each of manuka and pine to lift moods and balance emotions. Combine it with mandarin and geranium to soothe nerves and support mental clarity. In equal amounts with sandalwood, it helps foster a sense of well-being.

For energy work, manuka activates the sacral, solar plexus, and heart chakras. Use it to clear meditation space and to ground energy. It is also an aid when sending healing prayers. For candle magic, use manuka to remove any type of negativity and attract abundance.

For the Home

With its antibacterial, antiseptic, and antifungal properties, manuka works well for cleaning bath and kitchen surfaces and the laundry room. When work around the house, garden, or shop results in dirty hands, use manuka to scrub them clean.

Manuka Hand Scrub

¼ cup coarse sea salt

¼ cup sugar (brown or white)

3 tablespoons coconut carrier oil

10 drops manuka essential oil

6 drops lemon essential oil

5 drops peppermint essential oil

Combine the dry ingredients in a glass or ceramic bowl. Melt the coconut oil (if necessary) and add the essential oils. Mix all ingredients together. Store the mixture in a jar with a tight-fitting lid.

Sugar is added to the scrub recipe to soften the abrasiveness of the salt. If you have sensitive skin, use sugar without salt.

Manuka is known for its insect-repellent qualities. To boost its effectiveness and enhance the scent, combine manuka in equal amounts with eucalyptus (lemon) and lavender. For aromatic feng shui, use manuka to slow and calm energy in your home.

· · · · · · ·

✒ Marjoram ✑

BOTANICAL NAME: *Origanum majorana* syn. *Majorana hortensis*
ALSO KNOWN AS: Joy of the mountain, knotted marjoram, sweet marjoram

Reaching about twelve inches high, marjoram has gray-green leaves and numerous branches that give the plant a bushy appearance. The green buds look like knots until they open into spherical clusters of tiny white or pink flowers. This plant shares the nickname *joy of the mountain* with its close cousin oregano (*O. vulgare*).

Regarded as a sweeter version of oregano, marjoram was used by the ancient Greeks to treat arthritis and by the Romans for indigestion. Water scented with marjoram was used for bathing and for laundry. During the Middle Ages, marjoram was more popular than thyme in Britain, perhaps because both famous herbalists John Gerard and Nicholas Culpeper sang its praises in their books. Marjoram was used as a general strewing herb and for fumigating sickrooms. Not wanting to leave this herb behind, European settlers took it with them and introduced the plant into North America.

Oil Description and Precautions

Steam distillation of the flowers and leaves produces an oil that ranges from pale yellow to amber. It has a thin viscosity and an approximate shelf life of two to three years. Avoid using marjoram essential oil during pregnancy; use in moderation; may cause drowsiness.

Blending for Scent

This oil has a spicy, herbaceous scent with a slightly woody undertone. Some oils that blend well with marjoram include cedarwood, chamomile, eucalyptus, lavender, lemon, orange, rosemary, and thyme.

Scent Group	Perfume Note	Initial Strength	Sun Signs
Herbaceous	Middle	Medium	Aries, Gemini, Libra, Virgo

Medicinal Remedies

Marjoram is used for anxiety, arthritis, asthma, bronchitis, bruises, bursitis, chilblains, colds, constipation, coughs, headaches, indigestion, insomnia, lumbago, menstrual cramps, migraine, muscle aches and pain, nausea, premenstrual syndrome (PMS), sciatica, sprains and strains, and stress.

The antibacterial and antiviral properties of marjoram are an aid for coughs and colds to soothe inflamed mucous membranes. Use it in a steam inhalation or in a warm bath to help clear congestion. As an alternative, use 2 drops each of marjoram, thyme, and lavender in a tablespoon of carrier oil to make a warm compress for the chest.

For an effective massage oil to ease muscle aches and increase joint flexibility, combine 5 drops of marjoram, 4 drops of rosemary, and 3 drops of fir needle in an ounce of carrier oil. Marjoram's anti-inflammatory properties also help relieve temporomandibular joint pain (TMJ). When rubbed on the temples, this TMJ recipe is also effective for easing headaches.

Marjoram TMJ Relief

2 tablespoons carrier oil or blend

5 drops marjoram essential oil

2 drops rosemary essential oil

1 drop lemongrass essential oil

Combine all the oils, then gently massage the jaw muscles.

When dealing with symptoms of PMS, diffuse marjoram in equal amounts with chamomile and neroli. Alternatively, use these oils for a warm bath by mixing 6 drops of marjoram with 5 drops each of chamomile and neroli in an ounce of carrier oil. Relaxing and comforting, this bath blend is also helpful for getting restful sleep when diffused just before bedtime.

Personal Care and Well-Being

Mildly antiseptic, marjoram can be used as a toner for normal or combination skin. Mix 6 drops of marjoram, 5 drops of frankincense, and 2 drops of lemon in ¼ cup of cool chamomile tea. Marjoram also helps to improve a dull complexion. When dealing with dandruff, mix 5 drops of marjoram and 2 drops each of cedarwood and geranium in 2 tablespoons of carrier oil. Marjoram is also a good hair conditioner. Melt 1 tablespoon each of coconut oil and shea butter. Allow the mixture to cool to room temperature, then stir in 6 to 8 drops of marjoram. Refer to part 7 for details on working with butters.

Marjoram is a boon when it comes to balancing moods and lifting spirits, especially when recovering from bereavement. It also provides emotional support when coping with life's transitions. Diffuse 2 parts each of marjoram and bergamot with 1 part cedarwood. To combat nervous tension and fatigue, use the same proportions with fir needle and palmarosa. Marjoram also fosters a sense of peace and well-being.

When working with the chakras, marjoram activates the heart and third eye energy centers. In preparation for meditation and prayer, marjoram helps to ground and center energy. Use it in candle magic to attract happiness and love. Marjoram is also effective for dream work.

· · · · · · · ·

For the Home
For aromatic feng shui, marjoram is an aid to keep energy balanced. Diffuse a little or place a jar of marjoram salts in an area after you have stimulated or calmed the energy flow.

The Mint Oils

Plants in the mint family have the distinctive feature of square stems. While spearmint is considered the oldest species of mint, peppermint has been around for quite a long time too. Dried peppermint leaves have been found in ancient Egyptian burials. The Greeks and Romans valued both mints to help with digestive issues. The Greeks sprinkled spearmint leaves in bathwater for restorative soaks.

Both types of mints were introduced into England by the Romans. By the eighteenth century, peppermint and spearmint were widely used for medicinal and culinary purposes throughout Europe and North America.

✿ Peppermint ✿

BOTANICAL NAME: *Mentha* × *piperita*

ALSO KNOWN AS: Balm mint, brandy mint

Peppermint is a naturally occurring hybrid between spearmint (*M. spicata*) and water mint (*M. aquatica*). Its species name comes from the Latin word *piper*, "pepper," because its taste has a hint of pepper.[62] This popular garden plant reaches twelve to thirty-six inches in height. Its dark green leaves are deeply veined and toothed. Tiny purple, pink, or white flowers grow in whorls at the tops of the stems.

Oil Description and Precautions
Steam distillation of the leaves produces a pale yellow to greenish oil with a thin viscosity. It has an approximate shelf life of two to three years or slightly longer. Avoid using it during pregnancy; may cause skin irritation; avoid if you have high blood pressure; not compatible with homeopathic treatment; use in moderation; should not be used on children less than twelve years old.

Blending for Scent
The scent of peppermint essential oil is strongly minty and slightly camphoraceous. Some of the oils that blend well with it include eucalyptus, fir needle, juniper berry, lavender, lemon, mandarin, niaouli, pine, and rosemary.

62. Small, *Top 100 Food Plants*, 400.

Scent Group	Perfume Note	Initial Strength	Sun Signs
Herbaceous	Top	Very strong	Aquarius, Aries, Gemini, Virgo

Medicinal Remedies

Peppermint essential oil is used for acne, asthma, bronchitis, colds, constipation, coughs, depression, dermatitis, fainting, fever, flu, hangover, headaches, indigestion, inflammation, insect bites and stings, jet lag, migraines, motion sickness, muscle aches and pain, nausea, poison ivy, rashes, ringworm, scabies, sinus infection, stress, sunburn, and vertigo.

Peppermint is so effective for many applications because it contains menthol; spearmint does not. The menthol makes peppermint ideal for relieving chest and nasal congestion and most respiratory ailments. It is very effective in a steam inhalation. Read the information at the end of chapter 8 when using steam to relieve asthma.

An ointment made with peppermint can be used as an insect repellent or to soothe the swelling and itching of insect bites. It can be used to relieve skin irritation and rashes as well.

Skin-Soothing Peppermint Ointment

⅛ ounce beeswax

2 tablespoons apricot kernel oil

18–20 drops peppermint essential oil

Place the beeswax and carrier oil in a jar in a saucepan of water. Warm it over low heat, stirring until the wax melts. Allow the mixture to cool to room temperature before adding the essential oil. Adjust the consistency if necessary. Let the mixture cool completely before using or storing.

The ointment can also be used for scabies, or use peppermint in the bath. Combine 5 drops each of peppermint, lemongrass, and rosemary in an ounce of carrier oil, then add it to the tub.

A compress made with peppermint can reduce the inflammation and swelling of sprains and strains. To ease muscle pain, combine 3 drops each of peppermint, chamomile (German), and vetiver in a tablespoon of carrier oil. For headache relief, mix a drop of peppermint with a teaspoon of carrier oil and use it to massage the temples. To enhance and boost relief, add a drop of lavender. To cool heat rash, use 1 drop each of peppermint, clary sage, and tea tree in a tablespoon of carrier oil.

Personal Care and Well-Being

The antiseptic and astringent properties of peppermint make it a good choice for oily skin or the occasional pimple outbreak on normal skin. Make a facial scrub by combining 1 teaspoon of finely ground oatmeal with 2 or 3 drops of carrier oil and 1 or 2 drops of peppermint. Apply gently and rinse well with warm water. Peppermint also brightens a dull complexion.

To soothe sunburn or minor skin irritations, make a spray with 2 ounces of water, ½ teaspoon of carrier oil, 2 drops of peppermint, and 2 drops each of lavender and chamomile (Roman). Combine the ingredients in a spray bottle and shake well before each use. Alternatively, add 1 drop of peppermint to 2 tablespoons of aloe gel. Peppermint works well for an oily or dry scalp and helps control dandruff. It is also a good ingredient for deodorant.

Peppermint is instrumental in perking up the mind and emotions. Diffuse it in equal amounts with rosemary and lemon for help when dealing with major transitions and mental exhaustion. For energy work, peppermint activates the solar plexus, throat, and third eye chakras. Spiritually, it aids with healing prayers. Use peppermint in candle magic to attract luck and abundance. It is also helpful for banishing anything unwanted from your life.

For the Home

Peppermint can be used in a diffuser as an insect repellent, or make sachets with baking soda, lavender, and lemon for the linen closet. Combine peppermint with bay laurel to deter moths and a range of other insects. Place cotton balls with peppermint in an area where you suspect mice may be gaining access to your house. For aromatic feng shui, use peppermint wherever you need to get energy moving.

✍ Spearmint ✍

BOTANICAL NAME: *Mentha spicata* syn. *M. viridis*
ALSO KNOWN AS: Garden spearmint, green mint, lamb mint

The species name of this herb comes from the Latin word *spicate*, meaning "with spikes," which refers to the appearance of the flower stems.[63] Spearmint has tight whorls of pink or lilac flowers atop spikes with bright green leaves. Like peppermint, its leaves are deeply veined and toothed. Reaching twelve to eighteen inches tall, spearmint is the most commonly grown culinary mint. It is milder and less pungent than peppermint; spearmint is sweet, whereas peppermint has a sharp flavor.

Oil Description and Precautions

Steam distillation of the flower tops produces an oil that ranges from pale yellow to olive. It has a thin viscosity and an approximate shelf life of two to three years. Spearmint essential oil may cause dermatitis in some; may cause sensitization, especially in children; not compatible with homeopathic treatment.

---

63. Neal, *Gardener's Latin*, 115.

Blending for Scent

This oil has a minty, herbaceous, and slightly spicy scent that is less pungent than peppermint. Some of the oils that blend well with spearmint include basil, bay laurel, eucalyptus, lavender, lemon, lime, mandarin, niaouli, orange, and rosemary.

Scent Group	Perfume Note	Initial Strength	Sun Signs
Herbaceous	Top	Medium	Gemini, Libra

Medicinal Remedies

Spearmint is used for acne, anxiety, asthma, bronchitis, colds, coughs, dermatitis, fever, flu, hangover, headaches, indigestion, insect bites and stings, insomnia, menopausal discomforts, migraines, motion sickness, muscle aches and pains, nausea, sinus infection, sore throat, stress, and sunburn.

Although peppermint is a powerhouse with its menthol content, spearmint is also helpful for colds, especially if you want a gentler remedy. It has decongestant and expectorant properties that relieve coughs and ease congestion. Spearmint is also an antispasmodic, which soothes bronchial coughs. It can be used as a steam inhalation in the shower to chase away chills. Sprinkle 20 drops each of spearmint and hyssop on a washcloth, fold it in half twice, then place it on the floor of the shower under the water stream. Help bring down a fever with a cool compress prepared with 6 to 8 drops of spearmint in a quart of cool water.

To quell nausea, sprinkle a couple of drops on a tissue and inhale. Spearmint also helps when dealing with morning sickness. Put a drop or two in a cup of steaming water, then hold it near your face to inhale the vapors. For motion sickness, place 5 drops of spearmint and 2 drops of ginger in an inhaler to take with you on your travels.

Calming for the nerves, spearmint is also a sleep aid. Diffuse it in equal parts with chamomile before going to bed.

Personal Care and Well-Being

The antiseptic and astringent properties of spearmint fight acne on oily skin and work well for the occasional complexion blemish on normal and sensitive skin. As a splash-on face wash, it is especially nice on a hot summer day.

Cooling Spearmint Face Wash

4 teaspoons carrier oil

¼–½ teaspoon spearmint essential oil

2 cups water

Combine the carrier and essential oils. Swish into a bowl with the water and use your hands to splash it on your face.

Spearmint helps relieve an itchy scalp and deal with dandruff. Mix 8 drops in 2 tablespoons of carrier oil. Massage it onto the scalp, then wrap a towel around your head for about fifteen minutes before shampooing. To help combat foot odor, mix 6 drops of spearmint and 2 drops of grapefruit with a tablespoon of carrier oil. Swish it into a foot basin of warm water and soak until the water becomes cool.

The fresh scent of spearmint helps to lift mental and nervous fatigue. Put a few drops in a candle or diffuse it in equal parts with mandarin. For help in gaining mental clarity and dealing with changes, put 6 drops of spearmint, 3 drops of lemon, and 2 drops of bay laurel in an inhaler to waft under your nose as needed.

Use spearmint for energy work to activate the solar plexus, throat, and third eye chakras or for support during meditation and prayer. Spearmint helps attract love and luck in candle magic and supports dream work.

For the Home

Spearmint can freshen the air when used in a diffuser or deodorize a rug in a carpet powder. Combine 8 ounces of baking soda with 30 drops of spearmint or blend it with several other essential oils. Mix thoroughly with a fork to break up clumps. Lightly sprinkle the mixture over a carpet. Let it sit for thirty to forty minutes, then vacuum thoroughly. Spearmint also helps to deter insects and mice. For aromatic feng shui, use spearmint where you want to gently stimulate energy.

ᔐ Myrrh ᔑ

BOTANICAL NAME: *Commiphora myrrha* syn. *C. molmol*

ALSO KNOWN AS: Common myrrh, gum myrrh, hirabol myrrh

Aromatic gums and resins were a precious commodity in the ancient world. Along with frankincense, myrrh is one of the most famous. The word *myrrh* was derived from either the Arabic *murr* or Hebrew *mor*, both meaning "bitter" and referring to its bitter, pungent taste.[64] The genus name, *Commiphora*, means "gum bearing." [65]

Possibly the first to collect myrrh, the Egyptians used it for perfumery, medicine, and ritual. For thousands of years, it was used in Middle Eastern medicine, and like other resins, was regarded as a cure-all. As it was traded to the East, it was incorporated into the Ayurvedic med-

---

64. Foster and Johnson, *National Geographic Desk Reference to Nature's Medicine*, 256.
65. Quattrocchi, *CRC World Dictionary of Plant Names*, 596.

• • • • • • • •

icine of India. By 600 CE, myrrh had been introduced into China.[66] From ancient times to the Middle Ages, physicians sung its praises.

Native to northeastern Africa and the Arabian Peninsula, myrrh comes from a small shrubby tree with whitish-gray bark and thorny branches. It has small cream to yellowish flowers and leathery oval leaves that consist of three leaflets. The pale yellow resin exuded from fissures in the bark hardens to reddish-brown tear-shaped drops. It is still highly prized for incense and perfume.

Oil Description and Precautions

Steam distillation of the resin produces a pale yellow to amber oil. It has a medium viscosity and an approximate shelf life of four to six years. Avoid using this essential oil during pregnancy.

Blending for Scent

Myrrh essential oil has a bitter, spicy scent. Some oils that blend well with it include chamomile, clove bud, cypress, frankincense, lemon, palmarosa, rosemary, sandalwood, vetiver, and ylang-ylang.

Scent Group	Perfume Note	Initial Strength	Sun Signs
Resinous	Base	Strong to very strong	Aquarius, Capricorn, Pisces, Scorpio

Medicinal Remedies

Myrrh is used for arthritis, asthma, athlete's foot, blisters, boils, bronchitis, chapped skin, colds, corns and calluses, coughs, cuts and scrapes, eczema, hemorrhoids, indigestion, laryngitis, poison ivy, rashes, ringworm, sore throat, stretch marks, and vaginal infection.

The antifungal properties of myrrh help soothe ringworm and several other types of fungal infections. It can be used on its own, diluted of course, or combine 3 drops each of myrrh, manuka, and geranium in a tablespoon of carrier oil. To help reduce stretch marks, use 4 drops each of myrrh and elemi in a tablespoon of coconut oil. For boils and blisters, make a compress with equal amounts of myrrh and bergamot. Combine myrrh and lavender in an ointment to use as first aid for cuts and scrapes.

Before buying a commercial product for diaper rash, consider making your own. After all, do you really want to put something made with petroleum on your baby's bottom?

---

66. Foster and Johnson, *National Geographic Desk Reference to Nature's Medicine*, 256.

Myrrh Diaper Rash Gel

4 tablespoons aloe gel

8 drops myrrh essential oil

8 drops lavender essential oil

Mix ingredients well. Store in a jar with a tight-fitting lid.

Personal Care and Well-Being

Myrrh is ideal to hydrate dry or mature skin and combat wrinkles. For a basic moisturizer, combine 3 tablespoons of jojoba and 1 tablespoon of rosehip seed oil, 8 drops of myrrh, and 4 drops each of elemi and frankincense. For dry hair, use 2 tablespoons of coconut oil and 4 drops of myrrh to work through your hair before shampooing. To combat dandruff, massage your scalp with the mixture first.

Myrrh helps balance the emotions, lighten moods, and foster a sense of peace and well-being. Diffuse 3 parts myrrh, 2 parts cypress, and 1 part lemon. For support when dealing with major changes or grief, combine myrrh in equal parts with lemon balm. For mental clarity and focus, use it with rosemary.

When working with the chakras, myrrh activates the root, throat, third eye, and crown energy centers. Myrrh is especially potent for grounding and centering energy for meditation and when sending healing prayers. It is a powerhouse for purifying altars and areas used for spiritual practices. Use a few drops in a candle to express gratitude or to call on angels for aid. In candle magic, myrrh attracts abundance and success. It also supports past-life work.

For the Home

Enhance the scent of lemon oil furniture polish by adding 15 to 20 drops of myrrh to a 16-ounce bottle. For aromatic feng shui, use myrrh to balance energy.

Neroli
SEE *THE ORANGE OILS*

✌ Niaouli ✌
BOTANICAL NAME: *Melaleuca quinquenervia* syn. *M. viridiflora* var. *angustifolia*
ALSO KNOWN AS: Five-veined paperbark, paperbark tea tree, punk tree

Native to New Caledonia and the eastern coast of Australia, niaouli is a cousin to tea tree, eucalyptus, and cajeput. Usually growing thirty to fifty feet tall, the niaouli tree can sometimes reach eighty feet. Its whitish peeling bark looks like scrolls of paper. Its dark green leathery leaves have parallel veins, and its creamy white flowers resemble bottlebrushes.

· · · · · · · ·

For centuries, niaouli leaves have been used in traditional medicine to treat a range of ailments. After observing the locals, botanists sailing with Captain Cook took samples back to England. Niaouli oil was originally called *gomenol*, for the province of Gomen in New Caledonia, northwest of Australia, where it was distilled and exported.

Because of niaouli's remarkable similarity to the broad-leaved paperbark (*M. viridiflora*), it was originally classified as a variety of that tree. For a time, niaouli essential oil was called *MQV oil* because of its erroneous botanical name of *M. quinquenervia viridiflora*.

Oil Description and Precautions

This oil is produced by steam distillation of the leaves and young twigs. It has a thin viscosity and can be colorless, pale yellow, or greenish. It has an approximate shelf life of twelve to eighteen months. Niaouli is generally regarded as safe.

Blending for Scent

This essential oil has an earthy, herbaceous scent that is reminiscent of eucalyptus. Some oils that blend well with niaouli include bergamot, clove bud, eucalyptus, fennel, juniper berry, lavender, lemon, peppermint, pine, rosemary, and spearmint.

Scent Group	Perfume Note	Initial Strength	Sun Signs
Herbaceous	Middle	Medium	Leo, Scorpio, Virgo

Medicinal Remedies

Niaouli essential oil is used for acne, arthritis, asthma, boils, bronchitis, burns, circulation, colds, coughs, cuts and scrapes, fever, flu, headaches, insect bites and stings, muscle aches and pains, scars, sinus infection, sore throat, and whooping cough.

When packing a first aid kit for vacation, an antiseptic wash for disinfecting wounds is a good addition. Also keep it handy at home to treat backyard scrapes. Niaouli cleans as it fights bacteria and its analgesic properties help soothe pain. It can also help reduce scarring. The following recipe can be used as a spray or dabbed on the wound with a gauze pad.

Niaouli First Aid Wash

1 teaspoon carrier oil

15 drops niaouli essential oil

8 drops tea tree essential oil

7 drops helichrysum essential oil

4 tablespoons water

4 tablespoons distilled white vinegar

Combine the carrier and essential oils in a bottle, and then add the water and vinegar. Shake well before using.

Niaouli's antispasmodic properties help calm coughs. It also works as an expectorant, breaking up chest congestion. Use it to make a steamy healing shower. Put 20 drops of niaouli, 10 drops of pine, and 10 drops of hyssop on a washcloth, fold it in half twice, and place it on the floor of the shower under the water stream.

To ease a sinus infection, make a steam inhalation with 4 drops of niaouli and 2 drops each of cedarwood (Virginia) and eucalyptus. Diffuse niaouli to relieve colds and flu. For a sore throat, use it in equal parts with chamomile (Roman).

Personal Care and Well-Being

Like its cousins in the genus *Melaleuca*, niaouli works well for oily skin and hair, helping to balance oil production. To make a skin toner, mix ¼ cup of cool chamomile tea with 6 drops of niaouli and 4 drops each of bergamot and lavender in a bottle. Give it a good shake before applying with a cotton ball. For pimple outbreaks, mix 2 tablespoons of cool chamomile tea, 2 teaspoons of witch hazel, and 12 drops of niaouli to dab on the area.

Niaouli helps lift mental fatigue and focus the mind. To balance the emotions, diffuse 3 parts niaouli, 2 parts petitgrain, and 1 part rosemary. For energy work, niaouli activates the root, sacral, solar plexus, heart, and throat chakras. It is a supportive scent for meditation and spiritual practices, especially for sending healing prayers. In candle magic, use niaouli when you are seeking justice or when you need to banish negative energy.

For the Home

Niaouli helps to repel insects. Add a few drops to a citronella candle for outdoor dining or diffuse it in the home in equal amounts with lemongrass and lavender. Use a niaouli candle or salts for aromatic feng shui wherever you need to increase the energy flow.

The Orange Oils

Three essential oils from two types of oranges are included in this book. One is made from the peel of the sweet orange (*Citrus sinensis*) and two are made from the bitter orange (*C. aurantium* syn. *C. vulgaris*), neroli from the flowers and petitgrain from the leaves.

The sweet orange reaches twenty to forty feet tall and is believed to have originated in China. The bitter orange is smaller, ten to thirty feet tall, but hardier. It is also known as the Seville orange and sour orange. Both trees have oval evergreen leaves that taper at both ends and white five-petalled flowers. The bitter orange was the first type of orange introduced into Europe during the twelfth century.[67]

❧ Neroli ❧

BOTANICAL NAME: *Citrus aurantium* syn. *C. aurantium* var. *amara*

ALSO KNOWN AS: Orange blossom

Made from the flowers of the bitter orange, this oil was named in honor of Princess Anne Marie Orsini of Nerola, Italy. She adored the fragrance and made it all the rage throughout Europe in the seventeenth century. Symbolizing chastity, orange blossoms have been a mainstay of bridal bouquets for centuries. In North Africa and the Middle East, orange blossoms have been used as culinary and medicinal ingredients.

Oil Description and Precautions

Steam distillation of the flowers produces an oil that is pale yellow to coffee brown. It has a medium viscosity and an approximate shelf life of two to three years. Neroli is generally regarded as safe; it is not phototoxic.

Blending for Scent

This essential oil has a sweet, floral, and citrusy scent. Neroli blends well with chamomile, clary sage, coriander, frankincense, geranium, ginger, lavender, lemon, myrrh, palmarosa, rose, and ylang-ylang. The hydrosol by-product, which is a popular flower water, has a light, sweet floral scent.

Scent Group	Perfume Note	Initial Strength	Sun Signs
Floral	Middle	Strong to very strong	Aries, Leo

Medicinal Remedies

Neroli is used for anxiety, chapped skin, colds, constipation, depression, fainting, flu, headaches, inflammation, insomnia, jet lag, menopausal discomforts, premenstrual syndrome (PMS), scars, stress, stretch marks, and vertigo.

Famous for perfumery, neroli can do a lot more than make you smell great; its enchanting scent helps relieve anxiety and stress. Before taking a long soak in the tub, mix 7 drops of neroli, 6 drops of lemon balm, and 3 drops of patchouli in an ounce of carrier oil to add to your bathwater. For PMS, combine neroli with lemon balm and vetiver.

When dealing with depression, diffuse neroli in equal amounts with clary sage. For help in getting over jet lag, use 5 drops of neroli, 4 drops of rosemary, and 3 drops of ginger in an

---

67. Foster and Johnson, *National Geographic Desk Reference to Nature's Medicine*, 264.

inhaler. When feeling faint or experiencing vertigo, put a few drops of neroli on a tissue to inhale.

To reduce the appearance of stretch marks, melt together 1 tablespoon each of cocoa butter and olive oil. Allow it cool, then add 7 drops of neroli and 5 drops each of palmarosa and helichrysum. Mix well and let it set. (Refer to part 7 for full details on working with butters.) For chapped skin, combine a tablespoon of aloe gel with 2 drops each of neroli and palmarosa and 1 drop of myrrh.

Personal Care and Well-Being

Neroli works well on all types of skin and is especially good for dry, mature, and sensitive skin. It tones the complexion, improves elasticity, and helps reduce the appearance of thread veins and wrinkles. Use it as a moisturizer with frankincense and chamomile (Roman) in sweet almond carrier oil. For mature skin, use it with elemi and lavender in borage carrier oil. For oily skin, use neroli with lemon and cypress.

Neroli Deep Skin Moisturizer

2 tablespoons cocoa butter, grated or shaved

2½ tablespoons rosehip seed carrier oil

6 drops neroli essential oil

5 drops carrot seed essential oil

5 drops frankincense essential oil

4 drops palmarosa essential oil

Boil a little water in a saucepan and remove it from the heat. Place the butter and carrier oil in a jar in the water, stirring until the butter melts. Allow the mixture to cool, then repeat the process. When it cools to room temperature again, add the essential oils and mix thoroughly. Place the jar in the refrigerator for five or six hours. Allow it to warm to room temperature before using or storing.

For a scalp treatment to aid hair growth, combine a tablespoon of carrier oil with 2 drops each of neroli and rosemary and 1 drop of ginger. Because of its bacteria-fighting properties, neroli works well in a deodorant.

To ease nervous tension and calm the mind for sleep, diffuse 2 parts chamomile (Roman) and 1 part neroli before going to bed. Neroli fosters peaceful feelings and a sense of well-being. When you need to concentrate, combine neroli with basil or rosemary. To help maintain emotional balance, diffuse 3 parts neroli, 2 parts lemon, and 1 part basil.

When engaging in energy work, neroli activates the sacral, heart, and crown chakras. It is an aid for meditation and supports healing prayers and spiritual healing. For candle magic, use neroli to cultivate love and attract happiness.

For the Home

Neroli not only freshens the air but also kills bacteria that can cause nasty odors. It works well on carpets too. For a linen or storage closet, combine neroli with cedarwood to help keep moths away. Combine 15 drops of each essential oil and mix thoroughly with a cup of baking soda. Put it in a decorative container in the closet. For aromatic feng shui, use neroli wherever you need to slow and calm the energy.

ꙮ Orange ꙮ

BOTANICAL NAME: *Citrus sinensis* syn. *C. aurantium* var. *dulcis*

ALSO KNOWN AS: China orange, Portugal orange, sweet orange

As mentioned, this orange is believed to have originated in China. Not surprisingly, its species name means "of China." [68] Introduced into Europe in the fifteenth century, Portuguese travelers and traders sang the praises of this bright, sunny fruit.[69] It became a fashionable luxury to have an *orangerie*, a special greenhouse in which to grow citrus plants in cooler climates. Not long after its introduction into Europe, the orange was adopted as an ingredient in mulled wine.

Oil Description and Precautions

Cold expression of the peel yields a yellow-orange to dark orange oil. It has a thin viscosity and an approximate shelf life of nine to twelve months. Orange essential oil is phototoxic; may cause skin irritation.

Blending for Scent

This essential oil has a sweet, citrusy scent. Other oils that blend well with orange include basil, black pepper, cinnamon leaf, clove bud, clary sage, eucalyptus, lavender, lemon, marjoram, myrrh, patchouli, sandalwood, and vetiver.

Scent Group	Perfume Note	Initial Strength	Sun Signs
Citrus	Middle to top	Strong	Leo, Sagittarius

---

68. Coombes, *Dictionary of Plant Names*, 56.

69. Foster and Johnson, *National Geographic Desk Reference to Nature's Medicine*, 264.

• • • • • • • •

Medicinal Remedies

Orange essential oil is used for anxiety, bronchitis, colds, constipation, coughs, fever, flu, headaches, indigestion, inflammation, insomnia, nausea, seasonal affective disorder (SAD), and stress.

Just as drinking orange juice for colds and flu can ease symptoms, so too can using orange essential oil. With its antiseptic properties, orange is ideal to diffuse in a sickroom to freshen and disinfect the air. To cool a fever, place 6 or 7 drops in a tablespoon of carrier oil and add it to a quart of tepid water to make a compress.

To relieve indigestion, especially after eating too much, dilute 2 or 3 drops of orange in a teaspoon of carrier oil and gently massage the stomach area. Massaging the stomach and abdomen in a clockwise (up on the right, down on the left) direction can help ease constipation.

Soothe the Tummy Orange Blend

6 drops orange essential oil

2 drops peppermint essential oil

1 drop black pepper essential oil

1 tablespoon carrier oil or blend

Mix the essential oils together and combine with the carrier oil. Store any leftover oil in a bottle with a tight-fitting cap.

A soak in the tub with aromatic bath salts promotes relaxation and aids in dealing with stress. Combine 5 drops each of orange and clary sage and 2 drops of clove bud with 4 tablespoons of carrier oil. Mix it thoroughly with 2 cups of Epsom salt.

Use orange essential oil in an inhaler before an important event to combat performance anxiety. To help with seasonal affective disorder, diffuse equal amounts of orange, ginger, and ylang-ylang.

Personal Care and Well-Being

Orange is especially helpful to revitalize an oily complexion. Make an astringent with ¼ cup of herbal tea, 1 tablespoon of witch hazel, and 7 drops each of orange, peppermint, and palmarosa. Mix all the ingredients in a bottle, shake well, then apply with a cotton ball.

Orange's anti-inflammatory and antiseptic properties are especially helpful for pimple outbreaks. For these episodes, make an astringent (as noted above) with orange, juniper berry, and geranium. Orange isn't just for the face; use it in the bath or massage for all-over toning.

The citrusy scent of orange helps to clear the mind and ease nervous tension. Put 1 or 2 drops of orange in a teaspoon of carrier oil, then use a dab to massage on each temple. When it comes to emotional balance, orange is reviving and uplifting, fostering a sense of peace and well-being. Diffuse 3 parts orange and 2 parts each of lemon and cinnamon leaf.

• • • • • • • •

For energy work, use orange to activate the sacral, heart, and throat chakras. Orange provides general support for meditation and spiritual practices. When used in candle magic, it aids in attracting prosperity, happiness, and love and in achieving success. Orange is also helpful for dream work.

For the Home

With its antiseptic and bacteria-fighting properties, orange is well suited for cleaning surfaces, especially for cutting through grease. Combine 1½ cups of white vinegar, ½ cup of water, and 18 drops of orange essential oil in a spray bottle. Shake well before each use. For an all-around vinegar cleaner, use equal amounts of orange, lavender, and eucalyptus. Orange also works well to freshen and deodorize the air and carpets. To combat pests, use it as a general insect repellent or where ants may be a problem. For aromatic feng shui, use orange wherever you need to get the energy moving.

✖ Petitgrain ✖

BOTANICAL NAME: *Citrus aurantium* syn. *C. aurantium* var. *amara*

ALSO KNOWN AS: Bigarade petitgrain, true petitgrain

From French meaning "little grains," the name *petitgrain* comes from a time when tiny, unripe oranges, also called *orangettes*, were used for making oil.[70] The earliest reference to petitgrain was in 1694 by French pharmacist Pierre Pomet (1658–1699) in his *Complete History of Drugs*.[71] While petitgrain essential oil is also produced from small unripe lemons, mandarins, sweet oranges, and other citrus fruits, petitgrain from the bitter orange is regarded as the best. It is used widely in perfumes, including the classic Eau de Cologne.

Oil Description and Precautions

The leaves and twigs of the bitter orange tree are steam-distilled to create an oil that ranges from very pale yellow to almost amber. It has a thin viscosity and an approximate shelf life of two to three years. There are no known precautions for this oil; it is not phototoxic.

Blending for Scent

Petitgrain has a woody, herbaceous, and slightly citrusy floral scent. Oils that blend well with it include bergamot, cedarwood, cinnamon leaf, clary sage, clove bud, geranium, juniper berry, lemon, palmarosa, rosemary, sandalwood, and valerian.

---

70. *Webster's Third New International Dictionary of the English Language*, 1,690.
71. Poucher, *Poucher's Perfumes, Cosmetics and Soaps*, 165.

Petitgrain sur fleurs, also known as petitgrain neroli, is a distillation of leaves, twigs, and flowers. The scent is an interesting middle ground between neroli and petitgrain. It is used mainly in perfumery.

Scent Group	Perfume Note	Initial Strength	Sun Signs
Spicy	Middle to top	Medium	Aries, Leo

Medicinal Remedies

Petitgrain is used for acne, anxiety, depression, headache, indigestion, insomnia, seasonal affective disorder (SAD), and stress.

To relieve a headache, especially one caused by eye strain, make a cool compress with 4 drops of petitgrain and 2 drops each of basil and lemon balm. Combine the essential oils in a tablespoon of carrier oil and add it to a quart of water. Soak a washcloth, then rest with it over your eyes. As an alternative, mix 2 drops of petitgrain and 1 drop each of chamomile and spearmint in a tablespoon of carrier oil to massage the temples.

To calm panic attacks, use an inhaler with 6 drops of petitgrain, 4 drops of chamomile (Roman), and 2 drops of cedarwood (Virginia). For general anxiety, diffuse these oils in a 3:2:1 ratio, respectively.

When dealing with anxiety and stress, getting a good night's sleep can seem like an impossible dream as our minds run in overdrive, keeping us awake. A dream pillow placed nearby can help promote restful sleep. You can make your own little pillow or use a ready-made muslin bag.

Petitgrain Sweet Dreams Pillow

2 tablespoons dried lavender flower buds

2 teaspoons dried chamomile flowers

1 3 x 4-inch muslin bag

20 drops petitgrain essential oil

5 drops vetiver essential oil

Using a funnel, pour some of the dried flowers into the bag. Drip the essential oils onto a cotton ball, then place it in the bag. Use the funnel again to add as much of the remaining flowers as possible. Tie or sew the bag shut and store it in a plastic bag for a week to give the bag and cotton ball time to absorb the scents. When not in use, keep the pillow in the plastic bag to help it retain the scent.

Personal Care and Well-Being

As is the case with other citrus oils, the antiseptic properties of petitgrain work well for combination and oily skin. Combine it in equal amounts with juniper berry and lavender for a skin toner or moisturizer. For pimple outbreaks, combine a tablespoon of jojoba with 2 drops of petitgrain and 1 drop each of geranium and bergamot.

To condition oily hair, combine 2 tablespoons of coconut oil, 4 drops of petitgrain, 3 drops of cypress, and 2 drops of lemon. Petitgrain also works well in a deodorant and helps deal with excessive perspiration.

Aiding emotional equilibrium, petitgrain calms anger, reduces nervous tension, and fosters a feeling of well-being. Diffuse it in equal amounts with juniper berry and orange to promote mental clarity or recover from nervous exhaustion.

For energy work, petitgrain activates the solar plexus, throat, and third eye chakras. It is helpful for grounding and centering energy before meditation or prayer. In candle magic, it attracts good luck.

For the Home

Diffuse petitgrain wherever you need to freshen and deodorize a room. Alternatively, use it in a room spray or carpet powder. For aromatic feng shui, petitgrain helps keep energy in balance.

✍ Palmarosa ✌

BOTANICAL NAME: *Cymbopogon martini* syn. *C. martini* var. *motia*,
C. martini var. *martini*, *Andropogon martini*

ALSO KNOWN AS: East Indian geranium grass, Indian rosha, rosha oil, Turkish geranium

Cousin to lemongrass and citronella, palmarosa is a wild herbaceous grass indigenous to India and Pakistan that is now cultivated in some areas. Reaching six to nine feet tall, it has long, slender leaves and erect tufted stems with flowering tops. The words *Indian* and *Turkish* in its various names date to a time when the trade route for this plant was from Mumbai, India, to Istanbul, Turkey. The word *geranium* became part of its name too, because of its similar scent. The name *martini* is often spelled with two *i*'s at the end. For centuries, palmarosa has been used for culinary and medicinal purposes. Because of its rosy scent, it has been used as a substitute for and to adulterate otto (oil) of rose.

Oil Description and Precautions

Steam or water distillation of the leaves produces an oil that ranges from pale yellow to olive green. It has a thin viscosity and an approximate shelf life of two to three years. Palmarosa is generally regarded as safe; low risk of causing skin sensitization.

· · · · · · ·

Blending for Scent

Palmarosa has a sweet, floral, and rose-like scent. Some oils that blend well with it include bergamot, cedarwood, geranium, lavender, lemon, lemongrass, neroli, orange, rosemary, sandalwood, and ylang-ylang.

Scent Group	Perfume Note	Initial Strength	Sun Signs
Floral	Middle	Strong	Cancer, Pisces

Medicinal Remedies

Palmarosa is used for acne, anxiety, athlete's foot, bruises, chapped skin, dermatitis, eczema, fever, menopausal discomfort, premenstrual syndrome (PMS), rashes, scars, stress, stretch marks, and vaginal infection.

In addition to its popularity in perfume, palmarosa is a favorite for taking care of skin problems. The following ointment can be used for dermatitis and eczema and for general rashes. The recipe contains amounts for a 1% dilution, which is generally regarded as safe for use on the face. For use on the body, the amount of essential oils can be doubled.

Palmarosa Skin Rash Ointment

¼ ounce beeswax

3 tablespoons carrier oil or blend

6 drops palmarosa essential oil

4 drops carrot seed essential oil

3 drops geranium essential oil

Place the beeswax and carrier oil in a jar in a saucepan of water. Warm it over low heat, stirring until the wax melts. Allow the mixture to cool to room temperature before adding the essential oils. Adjust the consistency if necessary. Let the mixture cool completely before using or storing.

When dealing with stress, combine 4 drops of palmarosa and 2 drops each of grapefruit and rosemary in a tablespoon of carrier oil. Use it to massage your temples, or use this combination of essential oils in a diffuser. To aid in relieving PMS symptoms, diffuse 2 parts palmarosa with 1 part each of bergamot and clary sage.

Personal Care and Well-Being

Palmarosa is hydrating and nourishing, making it especially helpful for dry or damaged skin. For dry or mature complexions, moisturize with 8 drops of palmarosa and 5 drops each of chamomile (German) and carrot seed in 4 tablespoons of carrier oil. To combat wrinkles, use 5 drops each of palmarosa, lavender, frankincense, and lemon in 4 tablespoons of borage or evening primrose carrier oil.

The astringent and bacteria-fighting properties of palmarosa make it helpful for oily skin, too. Use it with peppermint and orange to make an astringent. For acne or pimple outbreaks, combine it with chamomile and myrrh. To keep oils in balance, make a toner with palmarosa, chamomile (German), and fennel.

To help steady the nerves and deal with tension or exhaustion, rest with a compress over your eyes or forehead. Prepare it with 4 drops of palmarosa, 3 drops of lemon, and 1 drop of cardamom in a tablespoon of carrier oil in a quart of cool water. To alleviate mental fatigue or to clear the mind, combine palmarosa with an equal amount of cedarwood in an inhaler. Diffuse equal amounts of palmarosa, bergamot, and geranium to create a calm, peaceful atmosphere that fosters a sense of well-being.

For energy work, use palmarosa to activate the heart, throat, and crown chakras. Palmarosa supports meditation and spiritual practices. Use it to clear an altar or sacred space and to ground and center energy. Add a drop or two to the melted wax in a pillar or jar candle when sending healing prayers. For candle magic, palmarosa removes negative energy and anything that you no longer want in your life. Also use it to attract love.

For the Home

The antiseptic and bacteria-fighting properties of palmarosa are ideal to freshen and deodorize wherever it is needed. Use it along with lavender, lemon, or eucalyptus for a kitchen or bath surface cleaner. For the home or personal care, it is effective in repelling mosquitoes. For aromatic feng shui, use palmarosa wherever you need to moderate and slow down the flow of energy.

✍ Patchouli ✍

BOTANICAL NAME: *Pogostemon cablin* syn. *P. patchouli*

ALSO KNOWN AS: Patchouly, puchaput

Reaching two to three feet tall, patchouli is a bushy herb with hairy stems and fragrant bright green leaves. Its white flowers have a tinge of purple and grow at the base of the leaf stems. Its genus name comes from the Hindustani words for "leaf" and "green."[72]

Native to tropical Asia, patchouli was used medicinally throughout Asia and the Middle East. Arabian travelers stuffed pillows with the leaves for protection against illness and to promote longevity. Patchouli has also been regarded as an aphrodisiac. It gained notice in Europe during

72. Foster and Johnson, *National Geographic Desk Reference to Nature's Medicine*, 282.

the early 1800s because of the sachets of leaves that were tucked into shipments of handmade shawls to protect them from insects during their passage from India. This fragrance was the hallmark of authentic Indian silks, and more than a century later, it became *the* scent for the counterculture of the 1960s and '70s.

Oil Description and Precautions

Oil produced from steam distillation of the leaves ranges from amber to dark orange. It has a medium to thick viscosity and an approximate shelf life of four to six years. Patchouli is generally regarded as safe.

Blending for Scent

Patchouli has a herbaceous and rich, earthy scent that gets stronger and deeper as it ages. Fresh oil may smell slightly harsh before it has had time to mellow. Some oils that blend well with patchouli include bay laurel, bergamot, cedarwood, chamomile, clary sage, clove bud, geranium, lavender, mandarin, myrrh, neroli, palmarosa, rose, sandalwood, and vetiver.

Scent Group	Perfume Note	Initial Strength	Sun Signs
Woody	Base	Strong	Aquarius, Capricorn, Scorpio, Taurus, Virgo

Medicinal Remedies

Patchouli is used for acne, anxiety, athlete's foot, boils, chapped skin, cuts and scrapes, depression, dermatitis, eczema, fever, headaches, insect bites and stings, menopausal discomforts, menstrual cramps, scars, stress, and stretch marks.

Because of its antiseptic properties, patchouli can be used on cuts and weeping sores to prevent infection. It also helps to reduce scars and marks left by severe acne or boils. For a massage oil to help ease menstrual cramps, combine 3 drops each of patchouli, chamomile, and thyme in a tablespoon of carrier oil.

Patchouli is a good stressbuster for relaxing in the tub. If you are a shower person, make a pre-shower rub by combining 8 drops of rosemary, 6 drops of lemongrass, and 4 drops of patchouli in 2 tablespoons of carrier oil. Alternatively, diffuse 3 parts clary sage, 2 parts petitgrain, and 1 part patchouli.

Personal Care and Well-Being

Patchouli helps maintain suppleness in mature skin. For a rejuvenating moisturizer, use patchouli, elemi, and lavender in a mix of jojoba and rosehip seed carrier oils. For puffy eyes, make a cool compress with patchouli and carrot seed. With its astringent properties, patchouli helps to balance oils and works well for oily skin and hair. It also helps when dealing with dandruff. Use patchouli for a refreshing after-bath splash that also helps keep body odor in check.

Patchouli Body Splash/Spray

6 ounces water

1 tablespoon witch hazel

1 teaspoon carrier oil

1 teaspoon bergamot, patchouli, and lavender essential oils

Place the water and witch hazel in a spray bottle. Combine the essential oils in proportions that appeal to you, then mix them in the carrier oil. Add the oils to the bottle and shake well before each use.

The scent of patchouli has a calming effect that helps you deal with emotional turmoil, especially when coping with unexpected changes or grief. Place a drop of patchouli and carrier oil on one palm and lavender on the other. Rub your hands together, then cup your nose to inhale the scent. To help revive from nervous exhaustion and bring mental clarity, use the combination of patchouli and peppermint.

Instilling a sense of peace and well-being, patchouli is particularly helpful to ground and center energy for meditation or prayer. Patchouli can be used to activate an individual chakra or all of them. For candle magic, use patchouli to remove negativity or to let go of something in your life, especially when seeking justice. Also use it to attract happiness and love.

For the Home

Famous as an insect repellent, patchouli can be diffused with lavender and spearmint to keep mosquitoes at bay. To deter moths, add about 15 drops of patchouli to a cup of cedar chips. It is also effective for disrupting ant trails. To freshen and deodorize areas around the house, use a little patchouli in a room spray or diffuser. For aromatic feng shui, use it wherever you need to moderate, calm, and balance the energy flow.

❧ Pine ☙

BOTANICAL NAME: *Pinus sylvestris*

ALSO KNOWN AS: Forest pine, pine needle oil, Scotch pine, Scots pine

Typically growing thirty to sixty feet tall in parks and yards, Scots pine can reach a hundred feet in the wild. Growing in pairs, the blue-green needles are about three inches long. The gray or

· · · · · · · ·

light brown cones are also about three inches long and hang from the branches. The species name is Latin and means "of the woods or forests." [73] Pine is native to Europe, and various parts of the tree were used medicinally. It was introduced into North America during colonial times.

In addition to lumber, pine also yields turpentine, tar, and pitch. Made from the resin, pine rosin has been especially important for violinists and other musicians to "wax" their bows. In the past, after resin was removed from the needles, the needle fibers were loosened and used to make "wool" for stuffing mattresses and cushions. Pine wool was also used to make blankets and served double duty by repelling fleas and lice.

Oil Description and Precautions

The needles and twigs are steam-distilled, creating a colorless or pale yellow oil. It has a medium viscosity and a slightly oily texture. Pine has an approximate shelf life of nine to twelve months. Avoid using this essential oil with allergic skin conditions; avoid during pregnancy; avoid with high blood pressure; may cause skin irritation; do not use on children under six years old. That said, Scots pine is regarded as the safest pine oil for therapeutic purposes.

Blending for Scent

Pine has a fresh woody and slightly turpentine-like scent. It is often called *pine needle oil*. Other oils that blend well with pine include bay laurel, cedarwood, eucalyptus, juniper berry, lavender, lemon, niaouli, and rosemary.

Scent Group	Perfume Note	Initial Strength	Sun Signs
Woody	Middle to top	Strong	Aquarius, Aries, Cancer, Capricorn, Pisces, Scorpio

Medicinal Remedies

Pine is used for arthritis, asthma, bronchitis, circulation, colds, constipation, coughs, cuts and scrapes, flu, gout, hangover, head lice, laryngitis, muscle aches and pains, scabies, sciatica, sinus infection, sore throat, sprains and strains, stress, and tendonitis.

The antiseptic and antibacterial properties of pine make it a good choice during cold and flu season. For relief on the go, use 6 drops of pine, 4 drops of eucalyptus (blue), and 2 drops of bay laurel in an inhaler to help clear the sinuses. Pine combines well with eucalyptus for a chest rub to ease congestion. For an expectorant, use equal amounts of pine and lemon in a steam inhalation. To soothe laryngitis, make a steam inhalation with pine and bergamot or frankincense.

73. Neal, *Gardener's Latin*, 120.

When it comes to arthritis, pine and fir needle make a warming, woodsy combination. When sore muscles need something more, a liniment may be the answer. While rubbing alcohol is often recommended for the base of a liniment, it dries the skin and for some people it can be more of an irritant than is usually intended with a liniment. Witch hazel makes a good base because it contains a low amount of alcohol.

Woodsy Pine Muscle Liniment

1 teaspoon carrier oil

10 drops pine essential oil

6 drops fir needle essential oil

¼ cup witch hazel

Combine the carrier and essential oils in a bottle. Add the witch hazel and shake well before using.

To combat head lice, use 3 drops each of pine, lavender, and lemongrass in 2 tablespoons of carrier oil. Massage the scalp and work it through the hair. Wrap a towel around your head for about an hour, then shampoo and rinse well. Be sure to launder the towel in hot water. For dealing with scabies, use 6 drops each of the same essential oils. Combine them in an ounce of carrier oil, then add it to your bath.

Personal Care and Well-Being

Although pine is rarely used for skin and hair care, its bacteria-fighting properties help when dealing with excessive perspiration. Add pine, along with your other favorite fragrances, to a deodorant recipe. To help with foot odor, add 6 to 8 drops of pine to a tablespoon of carrier oil and swish into a foot basin of warm water.

The revitalizing scent of pine aids in dealing with nervous tension and exhaustion. Use it to perk up from mental fatigue or when you need mental clarity. Fostering a sense of peace and well-being, it helps balance emotional ups and downs. To relax, diffuse 2 parts lavender with 1 part pine.

For energy work, pine activates the heart, throat, and third eye chakras. Use it for grounding and centering energy in preparation for meditation and prayer. For candle magic, pine helps banish negativity, supports justice, and attracts prosperity.

For the Home

Pine is used in so many commercial products because it is a good bacteria buster. Use it with lemon and thyme to clean kitchen surfaces. As an air freshener, it eliminates odors. As an insect repellent, it is especially good for deterring moths. For aromatic feng shui, use pine wherever you need to shake up the energy.

✐ Ravintsara ✐

BOTANICAL NAME: *Cinnamomum camphora* syn. *C. camphora* CT 1,8 cineole

ALSO KNOWN AS: *C. camphora* ravintsara, false camphor

The chemical components of the essential oil produced from *C. camphora* vary depending on where the tree is grown. Although it is most famous for producing camphor, when it is grown in Madagascar, it has little to none. Instead, the essential oil is rich in the component called *cineole*, which is very healing and not harsh, as is camphor.

When plants have different chemical profiles (chemotypes), the oil produced from them is noted with the letters *CT*. The chemotype for ravintsara is *1,8 cineole*. The *1,8* is a technical part of the name that refers to the molecule in which the oxygen atom connects with the first and eighth carbon atoms.

Native to Japan and China, this tree was introduced in the mid-nineteenth century into Madagascar, where it closely resembled a native species that had been used medicinally for centuries. The name *ravintsara* was derived from Malagasy words meaning "good leaf," referring to the healing power of its leaves.[74] And thus the confusion began because of two trees that looked similar and had leaves that were used for healing. Disagreement on the jumble of names also adds to the confusion.

The name *ravintsara* was Latinized to *ravensara*. The species of tree native to Madagascar has the botanical names of *Agathophyllum aromatica* and *Ravensara aromatica*. At one point, a subspecies was named *R. anisata*, referring to its somewhat anise- or licorice-like fragrance, but it was later discovered to be one and the same as *R. aromatica*. According to other sources, the native tree was *R. anisata* and the newcomer (the camphor tree) was *R. armomatica*. Scholars and experts do not agree on what the essential oil is that is sold under the names *ravensara, A. aromatica,* or *R. aromatica*.

Essential oils produced from the bark and leaves of *C. camphora* (usually the variety *C. camphora* var. linalool) in China are known as *ho wood* or *ho oil*. Although ravintsara is sometimes called *ho leaf oil*, it is a misnomer.

---

74. Halpern, *The Healing Trail: Essential Oils of Madagascar*, 51.

· · · · · · · ·

Oil Description and Precautions

Steam distillation of the leaves produces a clear oil with a thin viscosity. It has an approximate shelf life of two to three years or slightly longer. Avoid using ravintsara during pregnancy; do not use on children under six years old; may cause skin irritation.

Blending for Scent

This essential oil has a woody eucalyptus-like scent with a slight hint of spice or pepper. Some oils that blend well with ravintsara include basil, cajeput, chamomile, helichrysum, lavender, lemon, peppermint, sandalwood, spearmint, and ylang-ylang.

Scent Group	Perfume Note	Initial Strength	Sun Signs
Woody	Top	Medium	Gemini, Libra, Scorpio, Taurus

Medicinal Remedies

Ravintsara is used for arthritis, asthma, bronchitis, chicken pox, cold sores, colds, coughs, flu, hay fever, insomnia, laryngitis, muscle aches and pains, nail fungus, shingles, sinus infection, stress, and whooping cough.

The antiviral properties of ravintsara aid in healing shingles and relieving the pain of its blistery rash. It also eases the itching of chicken pox and helps to speed the healing of cold sores.

Ravintsara Gel for Shingles

2 tablespoons aloe gel

5 drops ravintsara essential oil

4 drops geranium essential oil

1 drop clove bud essential oil

Combine the essential oils and aloe gel. Mix thoroughly. Store any leftover gel in a jar with a tight-fitting lid.

Working as an expectorant and opening the airways, ravintsara is especially effective for respiratory ailments. Try a steamy shower for coughs and bronchitis. Put 20 drops each of ravintsara and peppermint on a washcloth, fold it in half twice, and place on the floor of the shower under the water stream. For whooping cough, use an inhaler with 7 drops of ravintsara and 6 drops of clary sage.

The easy vapors method (from chapter 8) helps you cope with asthma. Boil a cup of water, add 1 drop of ravintsara, then gently waft the steam toward your nose. For soothing relief from laryngitis, use a regular steam inhalation with 4 drops of ravintsara and 3 drops of eucalyptus

· · · · · · ·

(lemon). When the flu strikes, diffuse equal amounts of ravintsara and orange to clean and freshen the air of a sickroom.

Personal Care and Well-Being

The antibacterial properties of ravintsara help fight body odor. Combine it with lavender for a deodorizing body powder. Diffuse ravintsara when coping with nervous tension or nervous exhaustion. Its fragrance calms the nerves and fosters a sense of well-being. Combine it with peppermint to lift mental fatigue or focus the mind. It is also helpful when dealing with grief.

Ravintsara activates the energy of the sacral, solar plexus, heart, and throat chakras.

Grounding and uplifting, ravintsara is particularly supportive of meditation and spiritual practices. Also use it to prepare sacred space. Use ravintsara in candle magic to remove negativity and invite happiness into your life.

For the Home

Diffuse ravintsara to remove odors and the bacteria that causes them. Combine it with lemon for a fresh, clean scent. It is also an effective insect repellent against flies, moths, silverfish, and others. For aromatic feng shui, use ravintsara to keep energy in balance.

৩ Rose ৎ

BOTANICAL NAME: *Rosa damascena*

ALSO KNOWN AS: Bulgarian rose, damask or Damascus rose, otto or attar of rose, Turkish rose

Through the centuries, the rose has symbolized confidence, love, happiness, passion, and more. Its fragrance is recognized worldwide and has been written about throughout history. Linked with romance and allure, roses were also symbols of spirituality and mysticism.

Despite its name, the Damascus rose did not originate in Syria, the land of roses, but is thought to have come from Asia. This rose is a shrub that grows three to six feet tall. It has single medium-pink flowers and many thorns. This type of rose has been found in Egyptian tombs and is believed to have been introduced there during the reign of Ramses the Great (1279–1213 BCE). In Indian myth, Lakshmi, the wife of Vishnu, was found in a rose, and from this came the custom of a groom giving his bride attar of rose on their wedding day.

For centuries, rose oil has been known as otto of rose, rose otto, and attar of rose. When shopping for rose oil, it is common to find it listed under these names. While rose petals can be steam-distilled, this method has a low yield, making it expensive. Because rose absolute is often distilled into an oil, it is wise to use a vendor that offers specific information about the extraction methods for each oil. Rosewater hydrosol is the most famous floral water.

· · · · · · · ·

Oil Description and Precautions

A pale yellow or olive-colored oil is produced by steam or water distillation of the petals. It has a thin viscosity and an approximate shelf life of two to three years. Avoid using rose essential oil during pregnancy.

Blending for Scent

The scent of this oil is richly sweet and floral and just slightly spicy. Some oils that blend well with rose include bergamot, chamomile, clary sage, clove bud, geranium, lavender, myrrh, and patchouli.

Scent Group	Perfume Note	Initial Strength	Sun Signs
Floral	Top	Very strong	Cancer, Libra, Sagittarius

Medicinal Remedies

Rose is used for anxiety, asthma, bruises, chapped skin, circulation, depression, dermatitis, eczema, hay fever, headaches, inflammation, insomnia, menopausal discomforts, menstrual cramps, nausea, premenstrual syndrome (PMS), psoriasis, scars, stress, and stretch marks.

This beautiful flower can do more than symbolize romance; it's a powerhouse for skin problems and general care. For a bath to soothe the discomforts of dermatitis, eczema, or psoriasis, mix 8 drops of chamomile, 4 drops of carrot seed, and 3 drops of rose in an ounce of carrier oil before swishing it into the tub.

For healing bruises, mix 1 drop each of rose and lavender with 1 teaspoon of carrier oil. Gently apply it to the skin. This combination works well for stretch marks and scars, too. The anti-inflammatory properties of rose also help soothe chapped skin.

To help cope with depression, diffuse 2 parts rose with 3 parts each of clary sage and bergamot. For stress, diffuse it with mandarin and frankincense. Before bed, use rose with petitgrain and chamomile to encourage restful sleep.

Personal Care and Well-Being

While rose is appropriate for all skin types, it is especially good for dry, mature, and sensitive skin. In addition to moisturizing, it helps restore elasticity and refine skin texture. It also helps reduce thread veins and repair sun damage. Because the skin around the eyes is especially delicate, it is important to treat it with extra care. It can take a real beating from harsh eye makeup removers. Of course, the answer is to make your own eye makeup remover with rich, nourishing oils. Apply it with your fingertips and gently wipe off with a cotton pad.

Rosy Eye Makeup Remover

2 tablespoons coconut carrier oil

1 tablespoon rosehip seed carrier oil

8 drops rose essential oil

6 drops palmarosa essential oil

5 drops geranium essential oil

Melt the coconut oil, if necessary, and allow it to cool to room temperature. Add the essential and carrier oils and mix thoroughly. Store in a bottle with a tight-fitting cap.

The fragrance of rose provides a comforting atmosphere that helps reduce nervous tension and provides support when dealing with grief. To foster a sense of peace and well-being, diffuse 2 parts each of rose and mandarin with 1 part cedarwood. Rose also works well in combination with chamomile and peppermint.

For energy work, use rose to activate any chakra individually or balance all of them. This oil is especially effective to prepare an altar or meditation space. It supports spiritual practices, amplifies healing prayers, and is an aid for calling on angelic help. In candle work, use rose to attract happiness, love, and luck. It is also helpful for dream work.

For the Home

For aromatic feng shui, put 1 or 2 drops of rose in the melted wax of a pillar or jar candle wherever you need to balance the energy after stimulating or calming it. A room spray also works well.

℘ Rosemary ℘

BOTANICAL NAME: *Rosmarinus officinalis*

ALSO KNOWN AS: Compass plant, elf leaf, rosmarine, sea dew

Native to the Mediterranean region, rosemary is a shrubby plant with pale blue flowers and leaves that resemble pine needles. Often found growing on the sea cliffs of southern France, rosemary was described as having the smell of the ocean with a hint of pine. This is the source of its genus name, *Rosmarinus*, which is Latin, meaning "dew of the sea."[75]

In addition to using rosemary as a medicinal herb, the Greeks and Romans used it at weddings as a symbol of fidelity and at funerals for remembrance. In the belief that this herb improved memory, students in ancient Greece wore a sprig of rosemary in their hair for help in passing exams. In medieval Europe, rosemary blossoms were sugared and eaten as a preventive measure

75. Barnhart, ed., *The Barnhart Concise Dictionary of Etymology*, 671.

against the plague. At other times, this herb was burned in hospitals to fumigate rooms and clear airborne infections. It was also an important strewing herb that kept homes smelling fresh while repelling insects.

Oil Description and Precautions

A colorless or pale yellow oil is produced by steam distillation of the leaves and flower tops. It has a thick viscosity and an approximate shelf life of two to three years. Avoid using rosemary essential oil during pregnancy; avoid with epilepsy or other seizure disorders; avoid with high blood pressure; may irritate sensitive skin; do not use on children.

Blending for Scent

This oil has a minty, herbaceous scent with a woody undertone. Some oils that blend well with rosemary include bergamot, cedarwood, cinnamon leaf, clary sage, elemi, frankincense, geranium, lavender, marjoram, niaouli, petitgrain, pine, ravintsara, and thyme.

Scent Group	Perfume Note	Initial Strength	Sun Signs
Herbaceous	Middle to top	Strong	Aquarius, Aries, Leo, Sagittarius, Virgo

Medicinal Remedies

Rosemary is used for acne, arthritis, asthma, bronchitis, circulation, colds, coughs, cuts and scrapes, dermatitis, eczema, fainting, flu, gout, head lice, headaches, indigestion, jet lag, menstrual cramps, muscle aches and pains, scabies, sprains and strains, stress, tendonitis, varicose veins, and whooping cough.

To alleviate the chest and nasal congestion of colds, make a steam inhalation with 3 drops of rosemary and 2 drops each of sage and thyme. Diffuse rosemary on its own to help recover from chronic illness or ease a headache.

The warming analgesic effects of rosemary work well to relieve the pain and stiffness in the joints brought on by cold weather. Of course, soaking in the tub also helps relieve muscle aches and pains, and on a cold winter's night, there's nothing better for chasing away the chill.

Rosemary Warming Winter Bath

2 cups Epsom or sea salt

4 tablespoons carrier oil or blend

5 drops rosemary essential oil

4 drops marjoram essential oil

3 drops fir needle essential oil

Place the salt in a glass or ceramic bowl. Combine the carrier and essential oils and add to the dry ingredients. Mix thoroughly.

To ease the discomfort of varicose veins and aid circulation, use 6 or 7 drops of rosemary in a tablespoon of carrier oil for a massage. A drop or two of rosemary on a tissue is effective for reviving someone who has fainted.

Personal Care and Well-Being

Rosemary's antibacterial and astringent properties make it an ideal choice for oily skin, especially during pimple outbreaks. To help fade stretch marks, mix 5 drops of rosemary in a tablespoon of carrier oil and gently massage into the skin. Combine rosemary with a light carrier oil to massage into the scalp to get rid of dandruff and promote hair growth. Rosemary is also good for normal hair.

Use rosemary to balance moods, deal with grief, and promote general well-being. Like the students of ancient Greece who wore sprigs of rosemary, we can use its fragrance to improve concentration. For energy work, use rosemary to activate the root, solar plexus, throat, and third eye chakras.

Spiritually, rosemary can be used to consecrate an altar or sacred space or as a votive to support healing prayers. For candle magic, rosemary helps attract love and luck, banish negativity, and raise protective energy. It is effective when cultivating intuition and supports dream work and past-life work.

For the Home

The antibacterial and antifungal properties of rosemary make it a good choice for cleaning kitchen and bathroom surfaces. Combine ½ cup each of white vinegar and water in a spray bottle, add 10 drops of rosemary, and shake well. When used in a diffuser, rosemary freshens and cleans the air. It is also effective for pest control, especially mosquitoes. For aromatic feng shui, use rosemary to stimulate energy and get it flowing.

The Sage Oils

With hundreds of species of sage, it is easy to get them confused. Clary sage (*Salvia sclarea*) and Spanish sage (*Salvia lavandulifolia*) are included in this book. The essential oil of common sage (*Salvia officinalis*), also called *Dalmatian sage*, is not included. Because of its high level of the chemical component thujone, which is orally toxic and must be used with extreme care. Spanish sage is a good substitute because it has similar properties and no thujone. It is not harsh like common sage, either.

White sage (*Salvia apiana*), which is used as a sacred herb by Native Americans, is available as an oil but is not readily or reliably available as an essential oil. While blue sage essential oil is produced from plants commonly called *white sage* (*Artemisia douglasiana* and *A. tridentata*), they are not true sages and should not be confused with *S. apiana*.

✐ Clary Sage ✎

BOTANICAL NAME: *Salvia sclarea*

ALSO KNOWN AS: Clary, clary wort, clear eye, muscatel sage, see bright

Reaching two to three feet tall, clary has broad oblong leaves that are toothed and wrinkled. Whorls of small white and lilac or pink flowers grow on leafy spikes. Clary's species name is from the Latin word *clarus*, meaning "clear." [76] This comes from its centuries-long use for treating eye problems. In Germany, it was occasionally substituted for hops to brew certain types of beer and ale. Clary was sometimes called *muscatel sage* because it was added to cheap wine to give it a headier aroma like wine from Muscat grapes.

Oil Description and Precautions

The leaves and flower tops of clary sage are steam-distilled, producing a colorless to pale yellow-green oil. It has a thin to medium viscosity and an approximate shelf life of two to three years. Avoid using this essential oil during pregnancy and while nursing; avoid when taking sedatives or barbiturates.

Blending for Scent

Clary sage has a herbaceous scent that is both sweet and nutty. Some oils that blend well with it include cardamom, cedarwood, coriander, frankincense, geranium, juniper berry, lavender, and orange.

Scent Group	Perfume Note	Initial Strength	Sun Signs
Herbaceous	Middle to base	Strong	Aquarius, Libra, Scorpio

Medicinal Remedies

Clary sage is used for acne, anxiety, asthma, boils, coughs, depression, headaches, insomnia, laryngitis, menopausal discomforts, menstrual cramps, migraines, muscle aches and pains, premenstrual syndrome (PMS), rashes, sore throat, stress, and whooping cough.

While both clary and Spanish sage oils can be used for treating headaches, clary is the better choice because it is so calming to the nerves. It helps relieve tension, emotional turmoil, and stress, any of which can be the underlying cause of a headache. Combining clary with lavender and lemon balm creates an extra-soothing aroma. Diffuse the following blend or dilute the

76. Coombes, *Dictionary of Plant Names*, 176.

• • • • • • •

essential oils to a 1% ratio with carrier oil to rub on your temples. Mix it as a 2% dilution to dab on your wrists.

Clary Headache Relief Diffuser Blend
3 parts clary sage essential oil

2 parts lavender essential oil

1 part lemon balm essential oil

Combine the oils and then place them in the diffuser.

Clary also helps ease migraines. Diffuse it in any combination with chamomile (Roman), lavender, marjoram, and spearmint or mix it with carrier oil for a wrist rub. To ease PMS symptoms, clary works well with caraway seed or fennel. To soothe premenstrual cramps, combine 8 drops each of clary and palmarosa in 2 tablespoons of carrier oil for a massage oil. A warm compress with these oils also works well. To help with post-natal tension and depression, diffuse 3 parts clary sage, 2 parts rose or neroli, and 1 part bergamot.

To help soothe menopausal hot flashes, make a cool compress by combining 4 drops each of clary sage and spearmint in a tablespoon of carrier oil added to a quart of cool water. For night sweats, add 3 drops each of clary and spearmint to a tablespoon of carrier oil to massage the back of the neck and feet. To combat menopausal fatigue, put a drop each of clary and peppermint on a tissue and inhale.

The antispasmodic properties of clary sage soothe coughs and relax bronchial spasms. Combine 8 drops of clary with 4 drops of fir needle in an inhaler to use as needed.

Personal Care and Well-Being
Rich in antioxidants, clary is a boon to mature skin, tightening pores, improving skin texture, and reducing the appearance of wrinkles. It is especially helpful for the delicate skin around the eyes. Clary's antibacterial properties aid oily skin, combating acne as well as the occasional pimple outbreak. Make an astringent with ¼ cup of chamomile tea, 1 tablespoon of witch hazel, and 6 drops each of clary, bergamot, and spearmint.

Beneficial for dry, normal, and oily hair, clary sage makes a good conditioner. Combine 1½ tablespoons of coconut oil, 1 tablespoon of cocoa butter, 6 drops of clary, and 3 drops each of geranium and bay laurel. This hair conditioner is also good for split ends. Clary sage helps relieve dandruff and is a good deodorant ingredient to fight odor-causing bacteria.

Clary sage is particularly helpful for maintaining emotional balance and dealing with life's transitions. Diffuse 3 parts clary, 2 parts ylang-ylang, and 1 part cedarwood to lighten moods and foster a feeling of peace. To soothe nervous tension, combine clary with hyssop or mandarin and cypress. Clary with lemongrass and black pepper supports mental clarity.

For energy work, use clary to activate the sacral, throat, and third eye chakras. Use it when preparing for meditation and spiritual practices to deepen your experience. In candle magic, clary attracts happiness. It also aids dream work.

For the Home

Clary's antibacterial properties make it a good choice to deodorize the home. Combine it with lavender and neroli to freshen and scent linens. For aromatic feng shui, use clary to slow fast-moving energy and bring it into balance.

❧ Spanish Sage ❧

BOTANICAL NAME: *Salvia lavandulifolia* syn. *S. hispanorum*
ALSO KNOWN AS: Lavender-leaved sage, lavender sage, narrow-leaved sage,
Spanish lavender sage

The genus name for sage comes from the Latin word *salvare*, meaning "to be saved" or "to be safe."[77] Like its cousin common sage, Spanish sage is an evergreen shrub, but its grayish leaves are narrower and it has small blue-violet flowers. The whole plant is aromatic, with a fragrance similar to spike lavender (*L. latifolia*), which is more camphoraceous than true lavender. The species name *lavandulifolia* means "lavender-like foliage."

Native to the mountainous areas of Spain and southern France, this sage was regarded as a cure-all in Spain, where it was also believed to contribute to longevity. During the Middle Ages, it was used to guard against the plague. It is the type of sage most often used in Spanish cooking.

Oil Description and Precautions

Steam distillation of the leaves produces a pale yellow oil with a thin viscosity. It has an approximate shelf life of two to three years. Avoid using this essential oil during pregnancy and while breastfeeding; use in moderation.

Blending for Scent

Spanish sage has a fresh herbaceous, slightly pine-like, and camphoraceous scent. Other oils that blend well with it include bergamot, cedarwood, citronella, clary sage, eucalyptus, juniper berry, lavender, lemon, and rosemary.

---

77. Foster and Johnson, *National Geographic Desk Reference to Nature's Medicine*, 318.

Scent Group	Perfume Note	Initial Strength	Sun Signs
Herbaceous	Middle	Strong	Aquarius, Pisces, Taurus, Sagittarius

Medicinal Remedies

Spanish sage is used for acne, arthritis, asthma, boils, circulation, colds, coughs, cuts and scrapes, dermatitis, eczema, fever, flu, headaches, indigestion, inflammation, laryngitis, menopausal discomforts, menstrual cramps, muscle aches and pains, stress, and varicose veins.

Both clary and Spanish sage are effective for relieving muscle aches and pains. However, the anti-inflammatory properties of Spanish sage also bring warming relief for arthritis pain.

Spanish Sage Deep Relief Massage Oil

2 tablespoons carrier oil or blend

6 drops Spanish sage essential oil

4 drops rosemary essential oil

2 drops coriander essential oil

Combine the oils and mix thoroughly. Store any leftover oil in a bottle with a tight-fitting cap.

Make a similar massage oil using sage, cypress, and lemon to aid circulation and relieve the discomfort of varicose veins. Sage also eases indigestion when gently massaged on the stomach and abdominal areas.

During cold and flu season, sage helps to relieve chest and nasal congestion. Use 4 drops of sage, 3 drops of eucalyptus (blue), and 1 drop of thyme in a steam inhalation to clear the airways. In a diffuser, Spanish sage helps clean the air of a sickroom. Use equal amounts of sage and pine in a diffuser or steam inhalation to ease laryngitis.

Call on the antiseptic properties of sage for a first aid oil to treat cuts and scrapes. Combine 1 teaspoon of jojoba carrier oil and 1 drop each of sage, manuka, and orange. To relieve a painful boil, make a warm compress with 6 drops of sage.

Personal Care and Well-Being

Spanish sage is a tonic for keeping the scalp healthy. Use 4 drops in a tablespoon of carrier oil for a scalp massage. When dealing with dandruff, use 2 drops each of sage and lemon or lime. To encourage hair growth, combine sage with basil or cypress. If excessive perspiration is a problem, use sage in the bath or make a deodorant with lemongrass and petitgrain to fight body odor. It is also effective against foot odor.

Spanish sage helps keep emotions on an even keel, even when life throws you a curveball. Diffuse 2 parts sage and 1 part each of elemi and lime. For mental clarity and focus, use it in equal amounts with clary sage. To help cope with nervous tension and exhaustion, combine 7 drops of sage, 4 drops of palmarosa, and 3 drops of grapefruit in an inhaler.

For energy work, sage activates the throat and crown chakras. Its grounding scent is particularly helpful before meditation. Spanish sage is instrumental in spiritual practices for healing prayers and to express gratitude. In candle magic, use it to remove negativity and attract abundance.

For the Home

Diffuse Spanish sage or make a room spray to freshen and deodorize. It works well in a carpet powder too. Combine it with juniper berry and a little cedarwood to freshen closets. For aromatic feng shui, use sage wherever you need to tone down fast-moving energy.

Sandalwood

BOTANICAL NAME: *Santalum spicatum* syn. *S. cygnorum*

While the name *sandalwood* has been applied to various trees from several botanical families, trees from the *Santalum* genus are regarded as true sandalwood. Of these, *S. album*, or Indian sandalwood, is *the* sandalwood. Unfortunately, its popularity and overuse are causing its destruction, and it is considered a vulnerable species by the International Union for Conservation of Nature (IUCN). Don't despair, because the Australian government has been regulating the harvest of its sandalwood trees to ensure sustainability, and Australian sandalwood (*S. spicatum*) is becoming recognized for its own merits.

This tree reaches between ten and twenty feet tall and, like other sandalwoods, it has semi-parasitic roots. Its species name comes from the Latin word *spica*, meaning "spike," which refers to its narrow pointed leaves.[78] During the nineteenth century, the aromatic timber of Australian sandalwood was harvested to make incense mainly for the Chinese market.

Oil Description and Precautions

The roots and heartwood are steam-distilled, producing an oil that ranges from almost clear to light brown. It has a medium to thick viscosity and an approximate shelf life of four to six years. This essential oil may cause skin irritation or allergic skin reaction.

78. Boland et al., *Forest Trees of Australia*, 658.

Blending for Scent

The scent of this sandalwood is woody, somewhat balsamic, and slightly sweet. While it is more subtle than Indian sandalwood, it works well as a fixative for perfume. Oils that blend well with it include amyris, bergamot, black pepper, clove bud, geranium, lavender, myrrh, patchouli, rose, and vetiver.

Scent Group	Perfume Note	Initial Strength	Sun Signs
Woody	Base	Medium	Aquarius, Cancer, Leo, Pisces, Virgo

Medicinal Remedies

The chemical profile of Australian sandalwood differs from that of its Indian counterpart. While there has not been an in-depth study of this essential oil to determine its full therapeutic value, some of its properties are known and it is used for acne, boils, bronchitis, coughs, cuts and scrapes, insomnia, rashes, sinus infection, and stress.

Australian sandalwood has been found to be effective against the bacteria *Staphylococcus aureus*, which causes respiratory infections and skin rashes, particularly impetigo. Because of its bacteria-busting properties, sandalwood makes an excellent first aid treatment. The following ointment can also be used for boils and rashes.

Sandalwood First Aid Ointment

⅛ ounce beeswax

2 tablespoons sesame carrier oil

10 drops sandalwood essential oil

8 drops lavender essential oil

Place the beeswax and carrier oil in a jar in a saucepan of water. Warm over low heat, stirring until the wax melts. Allow the mixture to cool to room temperature before adding the essential oils. Adjust the consistency if necessary. Let the mixture cool completely before using or storing.

To help ease a sinus infection, use 3 to 4 drops each of sandalwood and ginger in a steam inhalation. Sandalwood's expectorant properties ease coughs, too. Diffusing it in a sickroom kills airborne bacteria.

Personal Care and Well-Being

Take advantage of sandalwood's astringent properties to control oily skin and fight pimple out-breaks. In a bottle, combine ¼ cup of your favorite flower water or herb tea, 1 tablespoon of witch hazel, and 8 drops each of sandalwood and bergamot. Shake well and use a cotton ball to apply. Sandalwood also helps to fight body and foot odor when used in the bath. It can make a nice addition to other scents in a deodorant as well.

Sandalwood helps bring emotions into balance. It fosters a sense of peace and well-being and is particularly helpful when dealing with grief and loss. For energy work, it can be used to activate individual chakras or balance all of them.

With its history of use as incense, sandalwood's grounding scent supports meditation and spiritual practices. Use it to consecrate an altar or sacred space. It can boost healing prayers and aid in contacting angels. For candle magic, use sandalwood to banish any form of negativity. It also attracts happiness, luck, and love. Sandalwood provides energetic support when seeking justice and for achieving goals. It also aids dream work.

For the Home

Sandalwood's bacteria-fighting properties make it valuable for cleaning. For a super surface cleaner, use 2 cups of water, 2 tablespoons of Castile soap, and 7 drops each of sandalwood and lemon. Combine all the ingredients in a spray bottle, then spray on surfaces and wipe off with a damp cloth. Diffuse sandalwood with clove bud and lavender to freshen and clear the air wherever odors are a problem. Sandalwood also works well to deodorize carpets. Place a sandalwood candle or feng shui salts wherever you want to moderate and calm the energy flow.

✒ Tea Tree ✒

BOTANICAL NAME: *Melaleuca alternifolia*
ALSO KNOWN AS: Narrow-leaved paperbark, tea tree

Reaching about twenty feet tall, tea tree is an evergreen with papery bark, needle-like foliage, and spikes of purple or yellowish-white flowers. Native to New South Wales, it is cultivated in other areas of Australia. From the Greek words *melas*, meaning "black," and *leukos*, "white," its genus name refers to the contrasting shades of its leaves and bark.[79] Its species name means that the leaves alternate along the branches.

For centuries, the Aboriginal people of Australia used this tree for a range of remedies. British captain and explorer James Cook called it *tea tree* when he saw them making a brew with the leaves. Regarded as the strongest natural antiseptic, tea tree was a standard item in Australian Army kits during World War II. As its use proliferated through the ranks of other armies, it became known as the "wonder from down under."

---

79. Foster and Johnson, *National Geographic Desk Reference to Nature's Medicine*, 354.

• • • • • • •

Oil Description and Precautions

The leaves and twigs are steam- or water-distilled, producing a pale yellowish-green or colorless oil. It has a thin viscosity and an approximate shelf life of twelve to eighteen months. Tea tree oil may cause sensitization.

Blending for Scent

This essential oil has a slightly spicy and camphoraceous scent. Oils that blend well with tea tree include black pepper, clary sage, clove bud, cypress, geranium, helichrysum, juniper berry, lavender, lemon, marjoram, pine, ravintsara, and rosemary.

Scent Group	Perfume Note	Initial Strength	Sun Signs
Herbaceous	Middle to top	Medium	Capricorn, Pisces, Sagittarius

Medicinal Remedies

Tea tree is used for acne, asthma, athlete's foot, blisters, boils, bronchitis, burns, chicken pox, cold sores, colds, coughs, cuts and scrapes, fever, flu, head lice, inflammation, insect bites and stings, jock itch, nail fungus, poison ivy, rashes, shingles, sinus infection, vaginal infection, warts, and whooping cough.

Effective against bacteria, fungi, and viruses, tea tree is practically a first aid kit in a bottle. It helps the body respond to infection. Clean a wound with 2 or 3 drops of tea tree diluted in a teaspoon of witch hazel. This can also be used to soothe an insect bite or bee sting.

For painful wasp stings, mix 2 drops of tea tree and 1 drop of basil in a teaspoon of witch hazel. For the swelling and itching of tick bites and to prevent infection, apply a drop neat. You may also want to contact your doctor. To keep mosquitoes at bay, combine ½ teaspoon of lavender and ¼ teaspoon each of tea tree and cedarwood in a teaspoon of carrier oil. Add this to a spray bottle with 6 ounces of water and 1 tablespoon of witch hazel. Apply to exposed skin before heading outside.

Like its cousins cajeput and niaouli, tea tree is effective for soothing respiratory ailments. It is also an antiseptic that can be diffused to freshen a sickroom and help reduce the spread of infection. Diffuse tea tree on its own or use 2 parts tea tree and 1 part each of pine and thyme. A couple of drops of tea tree in a teaspoon of carrier oil makes a quick and easy chest rub. Its expectorant properties make it effective for bronchitis and whooping coughs.

Personal Care and Well-Being

For skin care, tea tree helps to tone and balance oily skin and control pimple outbreaks. Used as a facial steam, it unclogs and cleans pores. Tea tree helps control dandruff and can be used in a deodorant to neutralize body odor.

• • • • • • • •

To support emotional balance and foster mental clarity, diffuse 1 part each of tea tree, clary sage, and cypress. For energy work, tea tree activates the sacral, solar plexus, and heart chakras. Use tea tree to clear the energy around a meditation altar and in candle magic to banish negativity.

For the Home

Tea tree's antiviral, antibacterial, and fungicidal properties can boost the effectiveness of homemade cleaners while it also freshens and deodorizes. Tea tree cuts through mold and mildew. The following recipe can be used as a tub and tile cleaner or for dishwashers. Avoid using it on marble, as it can cause damage. Test a small area of tile first.

Tea Tree Mold and Mildew Remover

1 cup water

1 cup vinegar

½ teaspoon tea tree essential oil

Combine the ingredients in a spray bottle. Shake well and spray on. Let it sit for a minute, then wipe off.

To repel insects, especially spiders, moths, flies, and silverfish, use the above recipe but double the tea tree to 1 teaspoon. Spray it where bugs enter your home. For aromatic feng shui, use tea tree in areas where you want to keep energy in balance.

❧ Thyme ☙

BOTANICAL NAME: *Thymus vulgaris* CT linalool

ALSO KNOWN AS: Common thyme, English thyme, sweet thyme, white thyme, wild marjoram

Reaching about a foot tall, this bushy Mediterranean herb has oval leaves and small pink to lilac or bluish-purple flowers that grow in clusters. Its genus name comes from the Greek word *thymos*, meaning "courage and strength." [80] The Greeks and Romans used this herb not only in cooking but also as a healing antiseptic. Thyme was an ingredient in a range of remedies and was used to fumigate homes to ward off infectious diseases. Although sources differ, it is generally believed that the Romans took it over the Alps into the rest of Europe and Britain. At any rate, it did not take long for thyme to become a universal staple in gardens and medicine chests.

80. Peter, ed., *Handbook of Herbs and Spices*, 297.

Oil Description and Precautions

Steam distillation of the leaves and flower tops produces an oil that ranges from clear to pale yellow. It has a medium viscosity and slightly oily texture. Its shelf life is approximately two to three years. Avoid using thyme essential oil during pregnancy; avoid with high blood pressure.

About Thyme Oils

It is important to know a little about thyme essential oils. The first distillation of thyme produces an oil called *red thyme*. This is because the color can be reddish, reddish brown, or reddish orange. Distilling the plant material a second time results in *white thyme*, which is clear or pale yellow.

As with several other essential oils, the chemical constituents of thyme vary widely depending on where it is grown. The types are designated with the letters *CT*, meaning chemotype. Thyme has about six or seven chemotypes, each with different therapeutic properties. The type included in this book, CT linalool, is gentler than the others and can be used by people who are sensitive to the stronger chemotypes.

Blending for Scent

This essential oil has a herbaceous and slightly sweet scent. Other oils that blend well with thyme include amyris, bergamot, clove bud, grapefruit, lavender, neroli, pine, rosemary, and spearmint.

Scent Group	Perfume Note	Initial Strength	Sun Signs
Herbaceous	Middle to top	Strong	Gemini, Libra, Taurus

Medicinal Remedies

Thyme is used for acne, arthritis, asthma, bronchitis, bruises, burns, cellulite, circulation, colds, coughs, cuts and scrapes, dermatitis, earaches, eczema, flu, gout, hangover, head lice, headaches, inflammation, insect bites and stings, insomnia, laryngitis, menopausal discomforts, menstrual cramps, muscle aches and pains, scabies, sciatica, sinus infection, sore throat, sprains and strains, stress, and tonsillitis.

Thyme is useful for a range of respiratory problems because its warming and drying properties aid in clearing congestion. During flu season, use it in a diffuser to disinfect a sickroom. Used in an inhaler, thyme can soothe the inflammation and ease the discomfort of sinus infections. To boost its potency, use 5 drops each of thyme, ravintsara, and peppermint. This combination works well in a steam inhalation, too. Thyme helps reduce the inflammation and irritation of eczema, dermatitis, and acne.

Healing Thyme Salve

½ ounce beeswax

3 tablespoons sweet almond carrier oil

2 tablespoons borage carrier oil

¼ teaspoon thyme essential oil

¼ teaspoon palmarosa essential oil

Place the beeswax and carrier oil in a jar in a saucepan of water. Warm it over low heat, stirring until the wax melts. Remove it from the heat and cool to room temperature before adding the essential oils. Adjust the consistency if necessary. Let the mixture cool before using or storing.

To relieve a tension headache, make a compress with 8 drops of thyme in a tablespoon of carrier oil in a quart of cool water. Place the compress on your forehead and temples or the back of your neck. For relief from a hangover headache, place a few drops of thyme on a tissue and inhale.

Personal Care and Well-Being

Used as an astringent for oily skin, thyme helps to control pimple outbreaks. Its antibacterial properties make it ideal for use in a deodorant. Combine 4 to 5 drops of thyme in a tablespoon of carrier oil for a cleansing scalp treatment that also aids hair growth.

When dealing with grief, use thyme to lift and balance the emotions. For energy work, thyme activates the root, throat, and third eye chakras. It helps to ground and center energy for meditation and works well to consecrate an altar. Diffuse it to support healing prayers. In candle magic, use thyme to attract happiness, love, and luck.

For the Home

Use thyme in a surface cleaner to remove bacteria. Combine it with bergamot or lemon for an extra-clean smell to freshen and deodorize anywhere in the home. It also helps to repel insects. For aromatic feng shui, use thyme wherever you need to get the energy flowing.

✺ Vetiver ✺

BOTANICAL NAME: *Vetiveria zizanioides* syn. *Andropogon muricatus*

ALSO KNOWN AS: Khus, vetivert

Native to southern India and Indonesia, vetiver is a tall tropical grass with erect stems and narrow leaves. Its species name means that it resembles wild rice.[81] With its thick network of long

81. Neal, *Gardener's Latin*, 135.

spreading roots and rootlets, vetiver has been used in India to protect soil from erosion. In the past, fibers from this long grass were woven for matting, baskets, and awnings. When dampened to bring out vetiver's scent, sunscreens and awnings also kept insects at bay. Hand-held fans woven from this grass served double duty for cooling and imparting a delightful soothing fragrance. This practice was quickly adopted by women in the southern United States when vetiver was imported to America in the nineteenth century.

Oil Description and Precautions

The roots are steam-distilled, producing an amber, olive, or dark brown oil. It has a thick viscosity and an approximate shelf life of four to six years. Vetiver is generally regarded as safe.

Blending for Scent

This essential oil has a rich woody and somewhat smoky scent with sweet undertones that deepen with age. Oils that blend well with vetiver include angelica (root), cardamom, clary sage, cypress, geranium, lavender, neroli, orange, patchouli, rose, sandalwood, and ylang-ylang.

Scent Group	Perfume Note	Initial Strength	Sun Signs
Woody	Base	Very strong	Capricorn, Libra, Taurus

Medicinal Remedies

Vetiver is used for acne, anxiety, arthritis, circulation, cuts and scrapes, depression, inflammation, insomnia, menopausal discomforts, muscle aches and pains, premenstrual syndrome (PMS), sprains and strains, stress, and tendonitis.

The anti-inflammatory and antispasmodic properties of vetiver help to warm stiff muscles and relieve the pain of arthritis. Create a soothing massage oil by combining 5 drops of vetiver, 7 drops of lavender, and 3 drops of juniper berry in 2 tablespoons of carrier oil. Regarded as an aphrodisiac, vetiver can be mixed with orange and ylang-ylang for a sensual massage blend to share with your partner.

For sprains and strains, make a cool compress with 3 drops of vetiver and 2 drops each of chamomile and bay laurel in a tablespoon of carrier oil. As a sedative, vetiver promotes restful sleep. About an hour before bedtime, diffuse 1 part vetiver with 2 parts each of lavender and neroli. As an alternative, mix 1 drop each in a teaspoon of carrier oil to massage on your wrists and the back of your neck.

Personal Care and Well-Being

The astringent properties of vetiver are ideal for oily and combination skin. Mix ¼ cup of peppermint tea, 1 tablespoon of witch hazel, 7 drops of vetiver, and 3 drops each of lemon balm and petitgrain. Vetiver protects and rejuvenates dry and mature skin and evens skin tone. For a quick and easy moisturizer, mix 4 drops each of vetiver, palmarosa, and frankincense with 4 tablespoons of coconut oil.

Before heading outdoors, call on vetiver's insect-repellent properties. Mix 4 drops of vetiver in ½ teaspoon of carrier oil and combine it with 2 ounces of water in a spray bottle. Shake well and spray on exposed skin. Mix vetiver with your favorite scents for a deodorant.

Regarded as the oil of tranquility in Sri Lanka and India, vetiver is well known for being calming and relaxing. When feeling restless, diffuse 2 parts vetiver with 1 part each of rosemary and mandarin. Vetiver helps release toxic emotions and foster stability. It also calms nervous exhaustion and tension. Use the following diffuser blend for general relaxation or for grounding and centering energy for meditation and spiritual practices.

Peaceful Vetiver Woodsy Diffusion

3 parts vetiver essential oil

2 parts cypress essential oil

1 part patchouli essential oil

Combine the oils before adding to the diffuser.

For energy work, use vetiver to activate the root, solar plexus, heart, throat, third eye, and crown chakras. Place a drop or two in the melted wax of a pillar candle during meditation to cultivate spiritual balance. Use vetiver in candle magic to attract abundance, luck, and love. It is also an aid for dream work.

For the Home

Called *moth root* in India, vetiver is especially effective for repelling moths, which is why it was a common practice to place pieces of the root among linens. Boost the power and enhance the scent of citronella candles for cookouts with a few drops of vetiver in the melted wax. Indoors, place reed diffusers near open windows to discourage insects from entering. For aromatic feng shui, use vetiver wherever you need to slow and calm the flow of energy.

✨ Ylang-Ylang ✨

BOTANICAL NAME: *Cananga odorata* var. *genuine* syn. *Uvaria odorata*

ALSO KNOWN AS: Ilang-ilang

The genus *Cananga* has two varieties called *genuine* and *macrophylla*, which produce two essential oils, ylang-ylang and cananga, respectively. Ylang-ylang has a more heady floral scent and is usually the preferred oil. It is an ingredient in Chanel No. 5 perfume.

• • • • • • •

The ylang-ylang tree is native to southern India, Malaysia, the Philippines, and other islands in the region. It is a tropical evergreen with glossy leaves. Its spectacular yellow flowers have drooping petals that are six to eight inches long. In addition to being a source of wood and fiber, the tree is grown as an ornamental in gardens.

Ylang-ylang essential oil is unusual in that it has several grades that are produced by fractionating or limiting the distillation time. This is accomplished by siphoning off oil in batches at certain intervals and leaving the plant material to continue distilling for up to fifteen hours. The highest grade, called *extra*, is removed after 1 to 1½ hours. It has the most depth and richness of scent. *Grade 1* is removed after four hours of distillation. Both extra and grade 1 are considered the best for therapeutic purposes and for scent. *Grade 2* is distilled for seven hours. Grades 1 and 2 are commonly used in cosmetics. *Grade 3* is distilled for ten hours and is generally used to scent products such as soap. The grade called *complete* can be distilled for the entire fifteen hours or it can be a mixture of grades 1, 2, and/or 3.

Oil Description and Precautions

A colorless to pale yellow oil is produced by steam distillation of the flowers. It has a medium viscosity and an approximate shelf life of two to three years. Ylang-ylang is generally regarded as safe; use in moderation; overuse can cause headache and nausea.

Blending for Scent

Ylang-ylang has an intensely sweet, floral, and slightly spicy scent. Some oils that blend well with it include bergamot, cardamom, clary sage, clove bud, coriander, fennel, lemon, lime, myrrh, petitgrain, rose, tea tree, and vetiver. Ylang-ylang works well as a fixative.

Scent Group	Perfume Note	Initial Strength	Sun Signs
Floral	Middle to base	Medium	Pisces, Taurus

Medicinal Remedies

Ylang-ylang is used for acne, anxiety, depression, insect bites and stings, insomnia, menopausal discomforts, premenstrual syndrome (PMS), seasonal affective disorder (SAD), and stress.

A nice steamy shower with ylang-ylang can help ease the effects of depression or seasonal affective disorder. Create a comforting atmosphere by diffusing equal amounts of ylang-ylang, bergamot, and ginger. To help with anxiety and stress, combine 1 drop each of ylang-ylang, chamomile, lavender, and geranium in a teaspoon of carrier oil. Rub it on your temples or wrists. When used just before bedtime, it aids in getting restful sleep.

Ylang-ylang is especially helpful in dealing with the discomforts and emotional ups and downs of menopause and PMS. Often, a long soak in the tub with bath salts can work wonders to soothe aches and calm tension.

Women's Time Ylang-Ylang Bath Salts

2 cups Epsom or sea salt

2 tablespoons baking soda (optional)

4 tablespoons carrier oil or blend

5 drops ylang-ylang essential oil

4 drops cypress essential oil

3 drops marjoram essential oil

Combine the dry ingredients in a glass or ceramic bowl. Mix the carrier and essential oils and add to the dry ingredients. Mix thoroughly.

Long regarded as an aphrodisiac, ylang-ylang's exotic scent can serve as the base for a sensuous massage oil. Experiment with varying amounts of ylang-ylang, amyris, and neroli to find the right combination for you and your partner.

Personal Care and Well-Being

While ylang-ylang can be used on almost any skin type, its ability to balance sebum production is especially good for combination and oily skin. Use it in equal amounts with chamomile (Roman) and mandarin to make an astringent, toner, or moisturizer. Balancing oil production is also helpful for a dry or oily scalp and dandruff. Make a scalp tonic with 4 or 5 drops of ylang-ylang in a tablespoon of carrier oil. Before shampooing, put a few drops on your fingertips and massage your scalp. Ylang-ylang also aids hair growth.

In addition to being well loved for perfumery, ylang-ylang is popular for supporting emotional balance and coping with change. Fostering a sense of peace and well-being, ylang-ylang calms nervous tension and soothes anger. Diffuse 3 parts each of ylang-ylang and cedarwood with 2 parts palmarosa.

For energy work, ylang-ylang activates the sacral, solar plexus, and heart chakras. Its uplifting scent provides support for meditation and spiritual practices. For candle magic, use ylang-ylang to attract happiness and love.

For the Home

Diffuse ylang-ylang or place feng shui salts wherever you need to moderate and slow the energy flow in your house. A couple of drops of ylang-ylang in the melted wax of a pillar or jar candle also works well for this purpose.

• • • • • • •

PART SEVEN

Carrier Oils and Other Ingredients

With very few exceptions, essential oils should never be used directly on the body without being diluted because they can cause irritation or other problems. Carrier oils are also called *base oils* because they serve as a base for essential oils. Most carrier oils have a light scent that is usually not as strong as that of the aromatic oils and generally does not interfere with the fragrance of essential oils. Carrier oils do more than form a base; they also have healing and therapeutic properties that work in concert with essential oils. This section explores twelve of the most commonly used carrier oils. Each profile includes the oil's common, botanical, and other names; historical and background information; and a description of the oil and its healing properties and approximate shelf life.

Two additional oils profiled in this section are infused oils, which are created by soaking plant material in a carrier. In the case of calendula and St. John's wort, flowers are used to create the oils. In addition to the properties of these two oils, details on the various methods for making infused oils and how to make your own are included.

Because carrier oils are not the only substances used with essential oils, information about other common ingredients is included. A description of the properties of aloe gel and instructions on how to harvest your own gel are provided, in addition to information on beeswax, cocoa and shea butter, and several other ingredients that I felt required more than a simple mention. Finally, if you like using flower waters, try your hand at making your own with the instructions in this chapter.

Carrier Oil Profiles

Carrier oils are produced from the fatty portions of plants. They easily absorb essential oils, which become diluted as they are dispersed throughout the carrier oil. While most carrier oils

• • • • • • • •

are produced from seeds, kernels, or nuts, a few, such as avocado and olive, come from fruit. If you or anyone who will use your blends or remedies has a nut allergy, avoid using carrier oils produced from nuts. Because carrier oils come from fatty plant matter, they can go rancid if not stored properly. Like essential oils, they should be kept in dark, airtight bottles, away from sun and artificial light.

Almond, Sweet

Botanical name: *Prunus dulcis* syn. *P. amygdalus* var. *dulcis*

While the cultivation of almonds began in central and southwest Asia, some botanists believe that the sweet almond was a natural hybrid of wild species from western Asia. These adaptable trees could grow in poor soil, and by 1700 BCE, they were being cultivated in the Middle East.[82] Although pricey, almonds were a popular part of European cuisine by the Middle Ages. Prepared in many ways for various dishes, sweet marzipan is a treat that still delights.

The word *dulcis* in the botanical name means "sweet."[83] This carrier oil should not be confused with the oil from the bitter almond (*P. amygdalus*), which is used in flavoring and as scent in cosmetics.

Produced from the nut kernel, almond oil is a very pale yellow, with a faintly sweet, nutty aroma. Rich in minerals, vitamins, and proteins, sweet almond is a light all-purpose oil that softens and nourishes the skin and helps it retain moisture. It can be used for all skin types and is especially good for dry or sensitive skin. It helps heal irritations and eczema, and because it absorbs slowly, it works well for massage. Almond oil works well on dry or oily hair and aids hair growth. It is gentle enough to use on children. Almond oil has an approximate shelf life of twelve months.

Apricot

Botanical name: *Prunus armeniaca*

Native to China and Japan, the apricot was a valuable trade item in ancient times, especially in India, where it has been popular for several thousand years. The fruit, bark, and seeds are still used in Chinese medicine. Apricots are sometimes fuzzy like their cousin the peach. They were introduced into Europe by Romans returning from the Middle East. The apricot's common

82. Rosengarten, *The Book of Edible Nuts*, 4.

83. Harrison, *Latin for Gardeners*, 145.

name was derived from the Arabic *al birqûq*, meaning "early ripe."[84] During the Middle Ages, apricots were imported through Armenia and became known as the Armenian plum. An early import into North America, apricots were being grown at the Spanish missions in California by the end of the eighteenth century. *P. armeniaca* is the most commonly cultivated type of apricot.

Oil is produced from the apricot kernel and has a faintly nutty aroma. Its color ranges from just a hint of yellow to pale yellow. Apricot oil has a light texture and is easily absorbed as it softens the skin. Rich in minerals and vitamins, it can be used on all skin types and is especially good for dry, mature, and sensitive complexions. With anti-inflammatory properties, apricot oil relieves irritated or itchy skin. It works well on dry and oily hair, too. Apricot oil has an approximate shelf life of six to twelve months.

❧ Avocado ❧

BOTANICAL NAME: *Persea americana*

ALSO KNOWN AS: Alligator pear, Spanish pear

Native to Mexico and Central America, the avocado has been cultivated for thousands of years. Archeological evidence shows that this fruit was used in Mexico as early as 8000–7000 BCE.[85] Sixteenth-century Spanish explorers encountered avocados in the markets of Peru and transported them to the Caribbean and Europe. By the seventeenth century, avocados had made it to the British Isles. After World War II, they were grown in the Mediterranean region.

The word *avocado* was an attempt by Spanish explorers to pronounce the Aztec name of the fruit, which meant "testicle," referring to the fruit's appearance.[86] It is called *alligator pear* because of its texture and shape.

A thick olive-green oil is produced from the avocado fruit. It has a sweet, nutty, and slightly herbaceous scent. Avocado oil is rich in essential fatty acids, proteins, minerals, and vitamins, most notably vitamins A and E. Highly penetrating, it hydrates and nourishes the skin. This oil is ideal for dry, mature, and sun-damaged skin. Its anti-inflammatory properties soothe dermatitis and eczema. Because of its heavy texture, it usually works best when mixed with a lighter carrier oil. Avocado nourishes dry hair, helps with dandruff, and aids hair growth. This oil has a shelf life of six to twelve months.

---

84. Toussaint-Samat, *A History of Food*, 583.
85. Nandwani, ed., *Sustainable Horticultural Systems*, 156.
86. Ibid.

❧ Borage ❧

BOTANICAL NAME: *Borago officinalis*
ALSO KNOWN AS: Bee bread, burrage, star flower

Borage is a bushy garden plant that is famous for its drooping clusters of blue star-shaped flowers that yield a fragrant honey. The Greeks used borage to flavor wine and for a range of medicinal purposes. Pliny called the plant *Euphrosinum* because it was said to bring happiness, although it may have been the wine speaking.[87] According to folklore, borage was believed to impart courage. In medieval times, it was used as a restorative drink to lift moods and break fevers. It is still used in herbal medicine for fever and skin conditions and as a mild antidepressant.

Obtained from the seeds, borage oil is pale yellow, with a light sweet scent. It is often mixed with lighter-textured oils. Rich in essential fatty acids, minerals, and vitamins, borage can be used on all skin types and is especially beneficial for dry or mature complexions. It is slightly astringent, helping to balance oily skin. Prized for skin care, it hydrates while improving elasticity. This oil helps reduce scarring and stretch marks and soothes the inflammation and irritation of dermatitis, eczema, and psoriasis. While it penetrates well, it can leave a slight oily feel on the skin. Borage has a shelf life of approximately six months.

❧ Coconut ❧

BOTANICAL NAME: *Cocos nucifera*

The coconut palm tree has been used for culinary and medicinal purposes worldwide for thousands of years. It was called the *tree of life* because of its many uses, especially providing food and drinkable water on small islands.[88] The oil was also used for lighting. It still plays a role in traditional medicines, such as Chinese and Ayurvedic, and is the subject of ongoing scientific research.

Called *coconut meat*, the white lining inside the nut is dried and pressed to extract the oil. There are two types of coconut oil on the market: refined, or fractionated, coconut oil (FCO) and unrefined, or virgin, coconut oil (VCO). The refined oil is odorless and colorless and has reduced healing properties.

Virgin coconut oil is pale yellow or whitish yellow, has a distinctive coconut aroma, and is a solid below 70°F/21°C. It works well when combined with a lighter oil. Coconut oil is rich in essential fatty acids, minerals, and vitamins and is appropriate for all skin types. It is especially good for dry or mature complexions and sun-damaged skin. Coconut's anti-inflammatory prop-

---

87. Bonar, *The MacMillan Treasury of Herbs*, 50.
88. Small, *Top 100 Food Plants*, 186.

erties help heal eczema, psoriasis, and dermatitis and reduce scarring. Coconut is also nourishing for hair. It works well on dry and normal hair and aids hair growth. Coconut oil is highly stable and has an indefinite shelf life.

❧ Evening Primrose ❧

BOTANICAL NAME: *Oenothera biennis*

ALSO KNOWN AS: Evening star, king's cure-all, night light, night willow herb

This prairie wildflower from North America has a rosette of large leaves at its base and an erect stem that can reach three to five feet tall. Although not a true primrose, it was so named because of its resemblance to the smaller native of England. Blooming only at night, evening primrose's fragrant yellow flowers produce clusters of oblong seed capsules. The common name *night light* comes from the slight phosphorescence of the blossoms, which emit a faint light that is visible on dark nights. Native Americans used the roots for a medicinal tea and various other parts of the plant for other remedies. English settlers used the lemon-scented leaves as a culinary herb before using it medicinally in the eighteenth century.

A pale to golden yellow oil is extracted from the seeds. It has a fine texture and a sweet, slightly nutty aroma. Evening primrose oil is full of vitamins, minerals, and essential fatty acids. It absorbs well as it hydrates the skin and helps it retain moisture. This oil is especially helpful for dry or chapped skin and helps rejuvenate a mature complexion. It also aids in healing eczema and psoriasis. Evening primrose oil has an approximate shelf life of six months.

❧ Hazelnut ❧

BOTANICAL NAME: *Corylus avellana*

ALSO KNOWN AS: Cob nut, English hazel

Native to Europe, hazelnuts were an important part of the diet for thousands of years. It had some medicinal uses in England, where it was commonly used in hedgerows. Derived from Greek and Anglo-Saxon words, respectively, the genus and common names refer to the shape of the husk that surrounds the nut, resembling a hood or bonnet.[89] The hazel tree was imported into the Americas in the seventeenth century. Small round nuts are called *cobs*. Larger nuts are mistakenly called *filberts*, which come from a different tree (*C. maxima*). That said, the names *hazelnut* and *filbert* are often used interchangeably.

Hazelnut oil is obtained from the kernel and has a slightly sweet, nutty aroma. This pale yellow oil has a fine texture and is easily absorbed into the skin. It contains a range of vitamins and

---

89. Rosengarten, *The Book of Edible Nuts*, 95.

• • • • • • •

minerals, essential fatty acids, and proteins. Hazelnut oil is appropriate for all skin types, and because it is slightly astringent, it helps balance oily skin. Soothing inflamed conditions, hazelnut oil also protects the skin. It works well as a hair conditioner, too. The shelf life of hazelnut oil is approximately twelve months.

✺ Jojoba ✺

BOTANICAL NAME: *Simmondsia chinensis*

ALSO KNOWN AS: Coffee bush, deer nut, goat nut, wild hazel

Found at higher elevations, jojoba is a desert shrub that can live more than a hundred years. Its fruit capsules contain one to three seeds, which are also called *nuts* and *beans*. Native Americans used the seeds for food and the oil for cooking and medicinal purposes. The Coahuila tribe of Mexico made a drink from jojoba seeds, which European settlers adapted as a substitute for coffee. Even though jojoba was imported into Spain in the eighteenth century, there was little commercial interest in the plant until the 1930s, when the oil was discovered to be a liquid wax and a good alternative to expensive whale oil.

Jojoba has a clear golden color, a softly nutty and slightly sweet aroma, and a light texture. It is a liquid at room temperature but solidifies at 50°F/10°C. Highly penetrating, it is particularly good for the skin because of its similarity to the body's natural oil, sebum. Rich in proteins and minerals, jojoba is appropriate for all skin types to moisturize, improve elasticity, and unclog pores. It also helps reduce the appearance of fine lines. It is an anti-inflammatory that soothes irritated skin. Jojoba is an aid for dry scalp and dandruff. It works well on normal and oily hair, too. Jojoba oil is highly stable and has an indefinite shelf life.

✺ Olive ✺

BOTANICAL NAME: *Olea europaea*

Slow growing and gnarly, olive was *the* fruit tree of ancient civilizations. Domesticated between 4000 and 3000 BCE in the Near East, it was a valuable source of food and oil.[90] The Greeks and Romans used the oil in many ways for preparing, cooking, and preserving food. It was also used in perfumes, soaps, and medicines, and in lamps for lighting. Associated with the goddess Athena, the olive tree came to symbolize peace, security, and wisdom. In Spain, olive oil was used to make Castile soap, which became the must-have luxury item of the eighth century. During the Middle Ages in northern Europe, olive oil was an expensive commodity used mainly by the wealthy.

90. Alcock, *Food in the Ancient World*, 87.

• • • • • • •

Oil is extracted from the fruit, and not surprisingly, it smells like olives. It has a dark greenish color and an oily texture. Because the oil is thick, it is usually mixed with a lighter one. To get the most for healing and beauty, buy extra-virgin cold-pressed oil. Olive oil is rich in minerals, vitamins, proteins, and essential fatty acids. It is best for dry or mature skin to nourish it and help it retain moisture. It soothes irritated skin and helps reduce scars and stretch marks. Used as a conditioner, it helps repair damaged hair and deal with dandruff. Olive oil has a shelf life of up to two years.

❧ Rosehip Seed ☙

BOTANICAL NAMES: *Rosa rubiginosa, R. moschata, R. canina*
ALSO KNOWN AS, RESPECTIVELY: Sweet briar rose, musk rose, dog rose

Rosehip seed oil is obtained from the fruit (rosehip) of three types of roses. The rosehip is also called a *haw* or *rose haw*. Rosehips have a long history of medicinal use and have been found at prehistoric sites where they may have been used as food and/or medicine. The sweet briar rose (*R. rubiginosa*), made immortal by Shakespeare in *A Midsummer Night's Dream*, is a European garden rose that has become naturalized in North America. The dog rose (*R. canina*) is a wild rose found along roadways and pastures. A sandy shore is another favored habitat that has earned it the name *beach rose*. Appreciated for its rich scent, the musk rose (*R. moschata*) has been cultivated for many centuries. Although its origins are murky, it is thought to have come from the Himalayan region.

As its name implies, rosehip seed oil is obtained from the seeds. Ranging from a pinkish tinge to a golden reddish color, it has a slightly earthy aroma and light texture and is easily absorbed. This oil is rich in vitamins, essential fatty acids, and anti-aging omega-3 and omega-6 fatty acids. Appropriate for all skin types, it is especially nourishing for dry or mature complexions. Rosehip seed oil reduces fine lines, thread veins, scars, and stretch marks. For acne-prone skin, it helps balance oils. Its anti-inflammatory properties aid eczema and psoriasis. Rosehip seed oil has an approximate shelf life of six to twelve months.

❧ Sesame ☙

BOTANICAL NAME: *Sesamum indicum*

Sesame is forever linked with Ali Baba's magical phrase "open sesame," possibly inspired from the way the seed pods suddenly pop open and sound like a springing lock. Sesame is generally regarded as the oldest oilseed plant, with the earliest evidence of its use dating back to approximately 3000 BCE in the Indus Valley of present-day Pakistan.[91] Domestication and cultivation is

91. Kiple and Ornelas, eds., *The Cambridge World History of Food*, vol. 1, 413.

believed to have started in that region and then spread throughout the Near East and Mediterranean. The earliest written reference comes from Egypt in 256 BCE and notes the medicinal use of the oil.[92] Also attesting to its early use, the ancient Sanskrit language used the same word for *oil* and *sesame*. In India and Babylon, the oil served as an offering in religious ceremonies. Sesame remains popular for cooking and adding flavor to foods.

A pale yellow oil is obtained from the seeds. It has a sweet, nutty aroma and a medium to thick viscosity. It is slow to absorb, leaving an oily film on the skin and making it good for massage. Sesame is rich in minerals and vitamins, especially vitamin E. It moisturizes and protects the skin, heals wounds, and repairs damage. With anti-inflammatory properties, sesame oil relieves itching and helps control dandruff. Sesame oil has an approximate shelf life of six to twelve months.

✌ Sunflower ✌

BOTANICAL NAME: *Helianthus annuus*

With a genus name that honors the Greek sun god Helios, the sunflower's large yellow-rayed flower heads track the sun's daily journey across the sky. While there are about eighty species of sunflowers, *H. annuus* is the quintessential variety that can grow over ten feet tall, with a flower head that can measure four to twelve inches wide. Indigenous to the North American prairies, it was used by Native Americans for a wide range of medicinal remedies, everyday food, dyes, and adornments. It was also considered a ceremonial plant, especially for war dances. By the time the European settlers arrived, sunflowers were grown as crops by settled tribes throughout a large part of North America.

Sunflower oil is obtained from the seeds. It is pale to golden yellow and has a slightly nutty aroma. The unrefined oil is high in essential fatty acids, minerals, and vitamins. It is particularly high in vitamins A, D, and E. Sunflower oil has a light texture and is easily absorbed. Moisturizing and softening, it is appropriate for all skin types. Sunflower oil heals and repairs sun damage and reduces scarring and fine lines. With anti-inflammatory properties, it soothes acne and eczema. Sunflower oil has an approximate shelf life of six to twelve months.

Infused Oils

A couple of popular carrier oils are not oils per se, but are oils infused with material from other plants. Infused oils are commonly used for cooking; rosemary and garlic oils are particularly popular. The infused oils included here are calendula and St. John's wort. The base oil in which

---

92. Kiple and Ornelas, eds., *The Cambridge World History of Food*, vol. 1, 414.

they are infused is usually sunflower. If you make your own, any base oil can be used. The texture, aroma, and shelf life are dictated by the base oil in which the flowers are infused.

⚓ Calendula ⚓

BOTANICAL NAME: *Calendula officinalis*

ALSO KNOWN AS: Marigold, pot marigold, poet's marigold, Scotch marigold

Although calendula is commonly known as marigold, it should not be confused with the popular garden flowers French and African marigolds, *Tagetes patula* and *T. erecta*, respectively. Native to southern Europe, the calendula flower has been valued for its medicinal and culinary applications. While the ancient Egyptians used it for healing, the Greeks and Persians favored it for flavoring and coloring food. Regarded as the poor man's saffron, it was used to color butter and thicken stews and soups during the Middle Ages. Today, calendula is commonly used in herbal medicine for its anti-inflammatory and antiseptic properties.

An oil infused with calendula flowers can range from light green to rich golden yellow, with an earthy aroma. It is especially good for dry or chapped skin, helping to soothe and soften it. Calendula can be used in first aid to treat cuts, burns, and sunburn. It also helps reduce the appearance of scars and thread veins.

⚓ St. John's Wort ⚓

BOTANICAL NAME: *Hypericum perforatum*

ALSO KNOWN AS: Rosin rose, sweet amber

Although considered a weed by some, St. John's wort has a long history in folk medicine. It was popular with the ancient Greeks and Romans for healing and maintaining good health. It has been used for a range of ailments, including the treatment of wounds. St. John's wort was also used to create various red and yellow dyes.

This plant's bright yellow star-shaped flowers grow in clusters. Although it was named for St. John the Baptist, because it blooms around his feast day of June 24th, this plant's use dates to earlier pagan summer solstice celebrations. The word *wort* comes from the Old English *wyrt*, meaning "plant" or "herb." [93]

An oil infused with St. John's wort has a rich red color and an earthy scent. It can be used in first aid to treat cuts, burns, and sunburns. It soothes eczema and psoriasis. Its anti-inflammatory properties help relieve aches and pains. St. John's wort may cause sensitization; avoid use before going in the sun, as it may increase photosensitivity.

93. Durkin, *The Oxford Guide to Etymology*, xxxviii.

How to Make Your Own Infused Oil

Infused oils can be made through cold or hot methods. Making a cold infused oil is an easier but slower process. The hot infused method works best with the tougher parts of a plant such as the roots, fruit, and seeds. The cold method works best with leaves and flowers, which tend to be more heat-sensitive. Since both oils included here are made with flowers, the cold method is better.

Calendula oil can be made with fresh or dried flowers. Use fresh flowers for St. John's wort oil. When gathering flowers, wait until the dew has dried but before the heat of the afternoon sets in. Gently cut the flowers from the plant.

Infused Oil Recipe

1 pint oil

¼ cup dried herb, crumbled

or ¾ cup fresh herb, chopped

Place the flowers in a glass jar and slowly pour in the oil. Gently poke around with a butter knife to release any air pockets. Leave the jar open for several hours to allow additional air to escape. If most of the oil gets absorbed, add a little more to cover the flowers. After you put the lid on the jar, gently swirl the contents. Place the jar where it will stay at room temperature for four to six weeks. Strain the oil into a dark glass bottle for storage.

Flowers left in the oil longer than four to six weeks may turn moldy. To make a stronger oil, put fresh flowers in a glass jar, strain the infused oil into it, and repeat the process of letting them soak. When using fresh flowers, check for any condensation in the bottle after it is stored. The moisture content of fresh flowers is released into the oil and can foster bacteria growth.

Other Commonly Used Ingredients

In addition to essential and carrier oils, being familiar with other ingredients included in recipes will help you make the best selection for remedies, personal care products, and home preparations. This section also includes basic details on how to work with some of these ingredients.

✒ Aloe Gel ✒

BOTANICAL NAME: *Aloe vera* syn. *A. barbadensis, A. vulgaris*

Aloe is a familiar houseplant that is often kept in the kitchen for first aid treatment of burns. It is a perennial plant with succulent leaves that can grow up to two feet long from a center base. Contained within the leaves, the gel is pale and translucent and has a slightly herby scent. A yellow juice called *bitter aloe* is exuded at the base of the leaves when they are cut. Unlike the gel,

· · · · · · · ·

this juice can be unpleasantly smelly. Bitter aloe is also found just under the skin of the leaves. Also called *latex*, it should not be used on the skin or ingested.

Harvesting the gel from an aloe plant can be a lot of work. Buying it is easier, but there are a few things to be aware of before heading to the store. Following several consumer lawsuits, an investigation of aloe gel found that several mass-marketed brands did not contain aloe vera. Read the labels. First, look for organic gel in order to avoid pesticides. Check for the terms *inner leaf* or *whole leaf*. Inner leaf indicates that only the aloe gel was used, while whole leaf may contain some of the bitter aloe. Also, check the ingredients for parabens, fragrances (which are usually chemically produced), and petrochemicals.

Some products may contain carrageenan, which is a substance derived from red seaweed and used as a thickening agent. Carrageenan is often used as a vegan alternative to gelatin. Another term you may see on the label is *stabilized*, which indicates the use of additives to prevent darkening of the gel and loss of potency. Additives often include citric acid (see later in this section) or ascorbic acid (vitamin C) as preservatives. It may also include potassium sorbate as a mold inhibitor. Potassium sorbate is a salt of sorbic acid that is found in some fruit. However, the commercial ingredient is usually chemically manufactured.

All is not gloomy. Some manufacturers are yielding to consumer demand for chemical-free products and developing processes to avoid the use of chemicals. With a little research, you can find a product with which you are comfortable.

Aloe gel is pale and translucent and has a fresh herby scent. Well known for healing burns, it is also good for cuts, hemorrhoids, and scabies. It makes an excellent base for a diaper rash ointment. Aloe gel is a moisturizer that can be used for most skin types, including oily. It can be used on the scalp to help bring dandruff under control. Aloe gel has an approximate shelf life of six months.

How to Harvest Aloe Gel

If you want to harvest your own aloe gel, you will need a leaf that is at least a foot long to obtain enough. Leaves are sometimes available in the produce section of supermarkets. Once you have your leaves, cut off the bottoms and tops. Prop them upright for a few minutes to let the bitter aloe drain out.

When you are ready to start working on a leaf, place it on a large cutting board. Using a sharp knife, cut off the spiny sides. Cut the remaining leaf into strips about five inches long and one inch wide, which will make the job more manageable. Like filleting a fish, carefully slide the knife under the skin (or rind) to remove it. You will be left with a block of gel. Cut it into smaller chunks and use a blender to make a puree. If it froths while blending, give it a minute to subside. The gel will last for about a week in the fridge.

• • • • • • •

❧ Beeswax ❧

Beeswax is a substance secreted by bees that they use to form the structure of their honeycomb. Since ancient times, people have used it for skin care. A solid at room temperature, beeswax is used as a base ingredient that regulates the consistency of ointments, salves, and balms. It also helps protect the skin from airborne allergens.

Beeswax is also used for candles, which are regarded as superior because they improve the air by neutralizing dust and odors. Over time, a candle made of pure beeswax often appears to develop a whitish film or a frosted look. This is a natural phenomenon called a *bloom* and it does not affect the quality of a candle. If you don't like the somewhat rustic appearance this may create, set the candle on a sunny windowsill for a while until the film goes away.

Beeswax is sold in the form of blocks, bars, and pellets. The pellets are also called *pastilles*, *pearls*, and *beads*. Blocks of wax can be grated like cheese, which makes it easier to measure and melt. Pellets are easy to use but can be pricey. I find it economical to buy beeswax in 1-ounce bars, which equals 2 tablespoons. To measure smaller amounts, cut the bar in half for ½ ounce or in half again. To make it easier to cut, place the beeswax bar in a plastic bag and set it in a bowl of hot tap water for about ten to fifteen minutes.

When purchasing beeswax, especially for skin care, look for filtered cosmetic-quality beeswax. Unfiltered wax contains some pollen, honey, and debris from the hive. Filtered wax doesn't contain these things. It also has less of an aroma, so it doesn't usually interfere with the scent of essential oils. Filtering also makes the wax mix more easily and evenly with other substances, such as carrier oils. When used for candles, filtered beeswax burns more evenly. The term *pure* or *100% pure* on the label means that it was not mixed with any other type of wax. When purchasing beeswax for use on the skin, make sure it is cosmetic or organic grade.

While beeswax starts out white, it picks up color from pollen and ends up anywhere from pale amber to yellow to butterscotch brown. Like honey, the color depends on the types of flowers the bees foraged. While further filtering can produce a whiter beeswax, bleaching with chemicals is often used to present a pristine appearance. Check carefully before buying white beeswax.

When used in medicinal or beauty care, beeswax protects the skin while also allowing it to breathe. It softens and helps hydrate it by keeping moisture in. With vitamins A and E, beeswax aids cell regeneration and is especially beneficial for dry and mature skin. It helps reduce the appearance of fine lines and wrinkles. With antibacterial properties, it can be used on oily skin, especially when dealing with acne or the occasional pimple outbreak. Beeswax is also appropriate for sensitive skin. In addition, it soothes hemorrhoids, heals chapped skin, and reduces stretch marks.

· · · · · · ·

Butters

While the nut butters we buy for our morning toast have a soft, creamy texture, cocoa and shea are hard butters; however, they are not as hard as beeswax. They are sold in blocks and sometimes jars and are easily grated. I find that scraping with a paring knife is a convenient way to prepare amounts for measuring. When purchasing these butters, read the label to make sure you are getting just the butter. Some products that are labeled cocoa butter or shea butter may contain paraffin, petroleum, lanolin, fragrance oils (not essential oils), and artificial dyes. Details on what to look for are noted in the section for each individual butter.

Unlike beeswax, butters melt at a lower temperature, but they need to be heated twice. When making a preparation, grate or shave off the amount of butter you need. Combine it with carrier oil in a glass jar. Bring a little water to boil in a saucepan, remove it from the heat, then place the jar in the water. Stir until the butter has melted. Set it aside and let it cool to room temperature. You may notice that it precipitates; particles or little lumps seem to float throughout the oil.

Boil the water again, remove it from the heat, and place the jar in the water. Stir the mixture until the particles disappear. Let it cool to room temperature again, then add essential oils. Place the jar in the refrigerator for five or six hours, then remove it. Allow the mixture to come to room temperature before using or storing. Occasionally, it may have a slightly mottled appearance. Nothing is wrong; this is the nature of the butters. While little particles may appear again, these melt on contact with skin.

✺ Cocoa Butter ✺

BOTANICAL NAME: *Theobroma cacao*

As expected, cocoa butter comes from the cacao tree. It is made from the seeds/beans and is an important ingredient in chocolate. The shelled seeds are ground into a liquid called *cocoa liquor*. The liquor is pressed to separate the fat, which is the cocoa butter, from the cocoa powder. Later in the process of making chocolate, the two ingredients are reunited. Although it is light in color, cocoa butter has a mild chocolaty scent. Cocoa butter is the basis of white chocolate, along with milk, sugar, and a few other ingredients.

Cocoa butter is used as a thickening agent in a range of commercial products. It melts at body temperature, but not as quickly as coconut oil does.

Unrefined cocoa butter is yellowish and has a chocolate scent and valuable nutrients. Refined butter is bleached and deodorized through chemical processes to remove the color and odor, which unfortunately also removes the nutrients. The unrefined cocoa butter may contain natural sediments that appear on the surface of the oil after it's melted. These can be removed by straining with a muslin cloth. Like beeswax, a bloom may occur on the surface of cocoa butter because of the fat content. It does not affect the quality.

• • • • • • •

Containing vitamin E and other vitamins and minerals, cocoa butter is an excellent moisturizer. It is especially good for dry, mature, and sensitive skin. It soothes burns and sunburn. With its healing properties, cocoa butter is an aid to chapped skin, eczema, dermatitis, and psoriasis. It also soothes a dry, itchy scalp and makes a good hair conditioner. Cocoa butter has a shelf life of two to three years.

❧ Shea Butter ❧

BOTANICAL NAME: *Vitellaria paradoxa* syn. *Butyrospermum parkii*

Shea butter is a natural fat extracted from the seeds of the West African shea tree. This gnarly tree with leathery leaves grows in wooded savannahs. It is also commonly known by the French name *karite tree*. The name *shea* was derived from the Senegalese name for the tree, *shétoulou*, which means "tree butter." [94]

For thousands of years, shea butter has been important in everyday use for its healing properties and for general skin care. The oil was also used for lighting, heating, and cooking. It was a valuable trade commodity for ancient Egypt.

Unrefined shea butter has a yellowish color and a nutty, smoky-like aroma. Refined shea butter is white and odorless and lacks the healing and nourishing properties. The unrefined butter is rich in vitamins A and E, essential fatty acids, and minerals. Nourishing as it hydrates, shea butter is especially good for dry or mature skin. It heals chapped, cracked skin and helps reduce or avoid stretch marks. Use it as a base for healing eczema and psoriasis and other inflammations of the skin. It soothes a dry, itchy scalp and makes a good hair conditioner. Shea also helps soothe insect bites and has been used traditionally as an insect repellent. Shea butter has an approximate shelf life of one to two years.

❧ Citric Acid ❧

Citric acid is an organic acid that occurs naturally in citrus fruits and a few other types of fruit. It is used as a food preservative, as a flavor enhancer to add a tart taste to foods and soft drinks, and as a cleaning agent. It is also called *lemon salt* and *sour salt* and is used for cleaning. Citric acid softens water and creates fizzy bubbles when combined with baking soda and water.

Available in powder or liquid form, citric acid can be found in the canning section of grocery stores or in pharmacies. The powdered form is used for bath bombs.

An important thing to know is that most citric acid on the market does not come from fruit. Instead, it is obtained by feeding sugar to black mold (*Aspergillus niger*), and then processing the

94. Goreja, *Shea Butter*, 5.

• • • • • • •

resulting fermentation using sulfuric acid. All is not lost because some small manufacturers are producing citric acid from non-GMO fruit and sometimes from sugar cane.

❧ Epsom Salt ❧

MINERAL NAME: magnesium sulfate

Epsom salt is a mineral compound named for the town of Epsom in England, where its healing properties were discovered in the seventeenth century. It is used for arthritis, bruises, inflammation, muscle aches and pains, psoriasis, and sprains and strains.

Epsom salt can be purchased in a grocery store or pharmacy. Check that it is USP (United States Pharmacopoeia) grade, as this has a higher quality control and is better suited for use in personal care. The type of Epsom salt sold in hardware stores is usually agricultural or industrial grade and not as pure as USP.

❧ Flower Water ❧

As mentioned in chapter 2, floral water, or flower water, is an aromatic by-product of the essential oil distillation process called a *hydrosol*. Flower water can be purchased or made at home. There are three methods for making it: infusion, cold infusion (also called *maceration*), and steam distillation. Whichever method you choose, gather flowers after the morning dew has dried and gently pull off the petals.

To make an infusion, place the petals in a Mason jar. Boil some water and let it sit for a moment before pouring it into the jar of petals. Use enough water to cover them. Put the lid on the jar, let the petals soak for three to four hours, then strain them out. The cold infusion is simpler. Place the petals in a Mason jar and add enough water to cover them. Put the lid on, let the petals soak for about twenty-four hours, then strain.

The steam distillation method is a little more complicated but is fun to experiment with. You will need a big stainless-steel pot—a stock pot or lobster pot works well—and two small glass or ceramic bowls. Place one bowl upside down in the middle of the pot to serve as a pedestal. Place the other bowl right-side up on the first one to act as a catch basin. Add flower petals and water to the pot. The water level should come just to the bottom of the top bowl. Put the lid upside down on the pot. This will direct the condensation into the catch basin. When the water begins to boil, turn the heat low. To quicken the condensation process, place ice cubes on top of the upside-down lid.

To make the process a little less messy, put the ice cubes in a big plastic bag. Place a paper towel on the lid of the pot and the bag of ice cubes on top. The ice cubes may need to be replaced a few times. After thirty or forty minutes, turn off the heat and let the pot cool before retrieving the catch basin. After it cools, store the water in a jar with a tight-fitting lid.

· · · · · · · ·

Flower waters made with one of the infusion methods will keep for a few days, even if stored in the fridge. When made by the steam method, they can last several months. Even when stored in the fridge, they can go bad, being mostly water. If a flower water becomes cloudy or smells "off," throw it away.

✌ Water ☙

With the explosion of bottled waters and home filtration products, it's no wonder we can get confused about the different types of water. This also creates a dilemma about the type of water to use in homemade preparations.

Standards for public or tap water are regulated by the Environmental Protection Agency (EPA). This water is treated, disinfected, and regularly tested. Filtered water is basically tap water with the chlorine removed (filtered out). It also has reduced lead. Spring water originates from an underground source that flows to the surface and goes through natural filtration. Standards for bottled spring water are regulated by the Food and Drug Administration (FDA).

Originating as ground water or tap water, purified water is treated by deionization, distillation, or reverse osmosis. Purified water must meet FDA standards where any remaining impurities must be reduced to an extremely low level. During the process, minerals are removed.

As its name suggests, distilled water has gone through the steam distillation process. When the water turns to steam, minerals, metals, and contaminants are left behind. It is a type of purified water.

This brings us to the question of what type of water to use in our medicinal remedies, personal care recipes, and home care preparations. My opinion is that whatever type of water you drink and cook with is the water to use for preparations. After all, if you feel safe putting it *in* your body, you should feel safe putting it *on* your body.

✌ Witch Hazel ☙

BOTANICAL NAME: *Hamamelis virginiana*
ALSO KNOWN AS: American witch hazel, spotted alder, winterbloom

The hallmark of this shrubby tree is its yellow flowers, which bloom in late autumn. Resembling crinkled ribbons, these spidery flowers on bare branches brighten the dull landscape. Native to eastern North America, witch hazel was used by the Cherokee, Chippewa, Iroquois, and other tribes to treat a range of ailments, and it didn't take long for European settlers to follow suit. The word *witch* in its common name comes from an Old English word that means "to bend," in reference to its pliant branches.[95]

---

95. Small and Catling, *Canadian Medicinal Crops*, 64.

As its name implies, witch hazel extract is created through the extraction process, which involves treating plant material with a solvent, usually alcohol. Witch hazel extract is made from the leaves and bark, which are high in tannins, giving it a highly astringent and drying effect. Extracts are often distilled once or twice to remove some of the tannins.

The witch hazel commonly available in pharmacies and supermarkets in the United States is a distillate made by steam distillation of twigs and branches. Although it is milder and does not contain tannins, it retains the plant's astringent properties. Basically a hydrosol, commercial witch hazel usually contains 14–15% alcohol, which acts as a preservative. This type of witch hazel has a shelf life of two or three years. Alcohol-free witch hazel is also available. It has a shelf life of approximately six to twelve months. The following information pertains to the witch hazel distillate.

Well known for its astringent and antiseptic properties, witch hazel is best suited for oily and acne-prone skin. When used on mature skin, be sure to follow it with a moisturizer; it may be too drying for dry skin. As an anti-inflammatory, it calms irritated skin, reduces puffiness around the eyes, and soothes hemorrhoids. It eases varicose and spider veins and helps reduce the swelling of sprains. Witch hazel is also helpful for cuts and scrapes, bruises, insect bites, eczema, and psoriasis.

SUMMARY

As we have seen, aromatherapy is about more than scenting the air. Throughout history, people have been fascinated with aromatic oils and have used them for spiritual and healing purposes and to make their environments smell nice. Following in ancient footsteps, we began with an exploration of creating perfumes. While the beauty of aroma is in the nose of the beholder, the perfume note and scent group methods for selecting oils provide a starting point for producing blends that are uniquely our own. These blends can be used or adapted when making beauty products, allowing us to create an ensemble of fragrance with which to surround ourselves.

We also learned how our sense of smell is intimately linked with memory and emotion. The use of scent supports well-being and enhances spiritual practices. Using these oils in conjunction with the energy of the chakras also contributes to overall well-being and health. With scented candles being an integral part of many practices, we also learned how to bring a little bit of magic into our lives with essential oils.

Moving beyond the olfactory application is the topical use of essential oils in healing remedies to fight infection, heal skin problems, soothe sore muscles, ease joint pain, and much more. In addition to their health care applications, many essential oils help us avoid the use of harmful chemicals in the home for cleaning, freshening, and pest control. Essential oils can also be used in the ancient Chinese practice of feng shui to modify the energy of our homes, which supports well-being.

As we have seen, a long list of essential oils is not necessary to make effective health remedies, personal care recipes, or household preparations. Like the herbalists who made "simples," we can enjoy and get the most from the essential oils that we like and have on hand.

APPENDIX

Conversions and Measurements

Following are conversion charts to aid you in measuring ingredients for your preparations. Although a measurement chart of essential oil drops is included, it is important to keep in mind that viscosity varies. The chart is based on a thin viscosity, because it is the most common. If you are working with an oil that has a medium or thick viscosity, you may want to do a drop test. Put one drop of thin oil and one drop of medium or thick oil on a plate to compare sizes, and adjust your measurements accordingly.

Approximate Drop Measurement

Drops	Teaspoons	Milliliters	Ounce
20–24	¼	1	
40–48	½	2	
80–100	1	5	⅙

Dilution Ratio Guide

Carrier Oil	1 teaspoon/ 5 ml	2 teaspoons/ 10 ml	1 tablespoon/ 15 ml	2 tablespoons/ 30 ml
Essential Oil (1%)	1–2 drops	2–3 drops	3–5 drops	6–10 drops
Essential Oil (2%)	2–3 drops	4–7 drops	6–10 drops	12–20 drops
Essential Oil (3%)	3–5 drops	6–10 drops	9–16 drops	18–32 drops

Dilution Ratios in 2 Teaspoons/10 ml of Carrier Oil

Ratio	0.5%	1%	1.5%	2%	2.5%	3%
Essential Oil	1 drop	2 drops	3 drops	4 drops	5 drops	6 drops

Measurement Equivalents: Fluid/Volume

Teaspoon(s)	Tablespoon(s)	Cup(s)	Ounce(s)	Milliliter(s)
1	⅓			5
1 ½	½		¼	7.5
3	1		½	15
	2	⅛	1	30
	3	⅙	1 ½	45
	4	¼	2	60
1 teaspoon + 5 tablespoons		⅓	2 ⅓	80
	6	⅜	3	90
	8	½	4	120
2 teaspoons + 10 tablespoons		⅔	5 ½	160
	12	¾	6	177
	14	⅞	7	207
	16	1	8	237

GLOSSARIES

Botanical Glossary

compound leaf: A leaf made up of small leaflets along a stem.

cultivar: A variety of plant that is developed and cultivated by humans rather than natural selection in the wild.

deciduous: A tree or woody plant that drops its leaves as part of an annual cycle.

florets: Tiny individual flowers that make up a larger flower head.

flower head: A dense, compact cluster of tiny flowers.

gum: A thick plant secretion that is water-soluble. This term is often applied to resin, which is not water-soluble.

gum resin: A naturally occurring mixture of gum, resin, and a small amount of volatile oil.

heartwood: The centermost wood in a tree trunk.

kernel: The inner and softer part of a seed, nut, or fruit stone. In cereal plants, it is enclosed within a husk.

oleo-gum resin: A naturally occurring mixture of gum, resin, and volatile oil.

oleoresin: A naturally occurring mixture of resin and volatile oil.

perennial: A plant with a life cycle of more than two years.

resin: A solid or semisolid secretion from trees that is not water-soluble.

rhizome: An underground stem that stores nutrients for a plant. It is often regarded as a type of root.

spike: A long flower-bearing stem without branches.

toothed leaf: A leaf with serrated edges.

umbel: A common flower-cluster structure with multiple stems radiating from a central stem. Although it can be round like a globe, it most often has the shape of an umbrella.

whorl: A circular or spiral growth pattern of leaves, needles, or flower petals.

· · · · · · · ·

General Glossary

absolute: A highly concentrated viscous liquid, solid, or semisolid product distilled from a concrete.

aromatic extract: A product obtained by solvent extraction containing both volatile and nonvolatile components.

aromatics: Plants that produce high amounts of essential oil and have strong fragrances.

astringent: A substance that dries and contracts organic tissue.

balm: A preparation with a very firm consistency that forms a protective layer on the skin.

balsamic: A scent that is sweet, earthy, and rich.

camphoraceous: A pungent, clean, and slightly medicinal scent.

carrier oil: A fatty plant extraction used to dilute essential oils. It is also called a *base oil* or *fixed oil*.

chemotype: A variation in the chemical components of a plant due to climate and location.

CO2 extraction: An extraction method, also called *supercritical CO2 extraction*, that uses liquid carbon dioxide to obtain essential oil.

cold-pressed: A mechanical method of oil extraction where no external heat is used during the process. It is also called *expression*.

diffuser: A device used to disperse essential oils into the air.

distillation: A method for extracting essential oil that uses steam or hot water to separate the water-soluble and non-water-soluble parts of plants.

enfleurage: A time-consuming and labor-intensive method of extracting essential oil from flowers using a fatty substance such as tallow or lard.

essential oil: The concentrated non-water-soluble extraction from plants obtained by distillation or cold-pressing. It is also called a *volatile oil* because it evaporates quickly.

expression: A method of oil extraction, also called *cold-pressed*, where no external heat is used during the process.

fixative: An oil that slows the evaporation of volatile essential oils.

fixed oil: Oil obtained from plants that are fatty and nonvolatile. Also called *base oil* or *carrier oil*.

flower essence: An infusion of flowers in water, which is then mixed with brandy. It should not be confused with a tincture or an essential oil.

flower water: A by-product of distillation that contains the water-soluble molecules of aromatic plants. These are also called *floral waters, hydroflorates, hydrolats,* and *hydrosols*.

fuller's earth: Aluminum silicate used to remove as much color as possible from food-grade vegetable oils.

herbaceous: An herbal grassy scent that is sometimes called a *green* fragrance.

hydrodiffusion: A distillation method of essential oil extraction where steam is forced into the vessel from above rather than below the plant material.

hydrosol: Traditionally called *floral water* (i.e., rosewater), a hydrosol contains the water-soluble molecules of aromatic plants. It is also called a *hydroflorate* or *hydrolat.*

infusion: A mildly aromatic product created by steeping plant material in water or oil.

liniment: A preparation for rubbing on the body to soothe pain and stiffness by creating a counter-irritant.

lipophilic: A property of essential oils that means they are readily absorbed by fatty oils and waxes. This property allows essential oils to be dispersed in carrier oils.

maceration: An extraction of medicinal substances from plants made by steeping them in cold water. Also called a *cold infusion.*

ointment: A preparation with a slightly firm consistency that forms a protective layer on the skin.

partially refined oil: An oil that has been put through processes that often include bleaching, deodorizing, and winterization to give it a longer shelf life.

phototoxic: A phototoxic substance can increase the risk of sunburn and skin damage when exposed to direct sunlight after it is applied to the skin. The effect can last twelve hours or more.

pomade: A perfumed fat obtained during the enfleurage extraction method.

refined oil: An oil produced to have no odor and very little to no color.

resin absolute: An absolute created from resin by a further extraction process using alcohol.

resinoid: A substance created by solvent extraction of resins, gums, balsams, oleo-gum resins, or oleoresins. It can be a viscous liquid, a solid, or semisolid.

salve: A preparation with a semi-firm consistency that forms a protective layer on the skin.

sitz bath: A method of bathing in which a person sits in shallow water up to the hips. It is also called a *hip bath.*

solvent extraction: A process that uses chemicals to obtain essential oil from plant material.

strewing herbs: Herbs that are scattered on floors to freshen the air, act as pest control, and make it easier to sweep away the detritus of everyday living.

unrefined oil: An oil that has not been put through various chemical processes to remove color, odor, and other natural properties.

virgin oil: The oil obtained from the first pressing of plant material.

volatile: A substance, such as an essential oil, that is unstable and evaporates rapidly.

water distillation: A method of extraction where plant material is completely immersed in hot water.

water-soluble: A substance that can be dissolved in water.

Medical Glossary

abortifacient: A substance capable of inducing the abortion of a fetus.

acute: A condition or disease with a rapid onset that lasts a short period of time.

analgesic: A substance that relieves pain.

anti-allergenic: A substance that reduces the symptoms of allergies.

antibacterial: A substance that fights the growth of bacteria.

antifungal: A substance that prevents fungal growth.

anti-inflammatory: A substance that reduces inflammation.

antiseptic: A substance that destroys infection-causing bacteria.

antispasmodic: A substance that relieves muscle spasms and cramping.

antiviral: A substance that inhibits the growth of a virus.

arthritis: The inflammation of one or more joints, accompanied by pain and stiffness.

asthma: A chronic lung disease that inflames and narrows the respiratory airways.

chilblains: The painful inflammation of small blood vessels in the skin when exposed to cold and high humidity.

chronic: A persistent condition or disease that is long-term.

dermatitis: A general term that describes the inflammation of the skin when it becomes red, swollen, and sore.

eczema: An inflammatory condition that causes areas of the skin to become red, rough, and itchy.

edema: A painless swelling caused by fluid retention under the skin.

fungal infection: A common infection of the skin caused by a fungus that includes athlete's foot, jock itch, ringworm, and yeast infections.

gout: A type of arthritis that occurs when uric acid builds up and causes joint inflammation.

hemorrhoids: A condition caused by dilated rectal veins. They are also called *piles*.

premenstrual syndrome (PMS): A term that refers to a wide variety of symptoms that may include mood swings, tender breasts, food cravings, fatigue, irritability, and depression.

psoriasis: A skin condition that causes itchy or sore patches of thick, red skin, accompanied by silvery scales.

rheumatism: A term that has been used informally for a variety of inflammation and joint pain symptoms. It is no longer used on its own medically to define a disorder or ailment.

rheumatoid arthritis: A type of autoimmune arthritis that causes pain, stiffness, swelling, and limited motion in the joints.

ringworm: A type of skin infection caused by a fungus.

scabies: A contagious and very itchy skin infection caused by the *Sarcoptes scabiei* mite.

• • • • • • • •

sciatica: Pain or numbness that runs from the lower back down the leg along the sciatic nerve pathway.

seasonal affective disorder (SAD): A type of depression that occurs during the same season each year. It most often occurs in winter.

sensitization: Unlike irritation, a condition where the skin becomes increasingly reactive or hypersensitive.

sprain: A stretch and/or tear of a ligament.

staph infection: An infection caused by the *Staphylococcus* bacteria.

strain: A stretch and/or tear of a muscle.

styptic: A substance that stops minor external bleeding.

temporomandibular joint pain (TMJ): A pain that occurs in or near the jaw joint, which is caused by a range of problems.

varicose veins: The name given to enlarged, twisted blood vessels that appear blue and bulging through the skin.

. . . .

BIBLIOGRAPHY

Alcock, Joan P. *Food in the Ancient World*. Westport, CT: Greenwood Press, 2006.

Anderson, Graham. *Greek and Roman Folklore: A Handbook*. Westport, CT: Greenwood Press, 2006.

Arrowsmith, Nancy. *Essential Herbal Wisdom: A Complete Exploration of 50 Remarkable Herbs*. Woodbury, MN: Llewellyn Publications, 2009.

Aftel, Mandy. *Essence and Alchemy: A Natural History of Perfume*. New York: North Point Press, 2001.

Barnhart, Robert K., ed. *The Barnhart Concise Dictionary of Etymology*. New York: HarperCollins, 1995.

Barrett, Judy. *What Can I Do with My Herbs? How to Grow, Use & Enjoy These Versatile Plants*. College Station, TX: Texas A&M University Press, 2009.

Başer, K. Hüsnü Can, and Gerhard Buchbauer, eds. *Handbook of Essential Oils: Science, Technology, and Applications*. 2nd ed. Boca Raton, FL: CRC Press, 2016.

Bedson, Paul. *The Complete Family Guide to Natural Healing*. Dingley, Australia: Hinkler Books Pty. Ltd., 2005.

Behra, Olivier, Chantal Rakotoarison, and Rhiannon Harris. "Ravintsara vs Ravensara a Taxonomic Clarification," *International Journal of Aromatherapy* vol. 11, no. 1 (2001): 4–7. https://doi.org/10.1016/S0962-4562(01)80062-X.

Bell, Kristen Leigh. *Holistic Aromatherapy for Animals: A Comprehensive Guide to the Use of Essential Oils and Hydrosols with Animals*. Forres, Scotland: Findhorn Press, 2002.

Bennet, Doug, and Tim Tiner. *The Wild Woods Guide: From Minnesota to Maine, the Nature and Lore of the Great North Woods*. New York: HarperCollins, 2003.

Berens, E. M. *The Myths and Legends of Ancient Greece and Rome*. London: Blackie & Son, 1880.

Binney, Ruth. *The Gardener's Wise Words and Country Ways*. Newton Abbot, England: David and Charles, 2007.

Boddy, Kasia. *Geranium*. London: Reaktion Books Ltd., 2013.

• • • • • • • •

Bibliography

Boland, D. J., M. I. H. Brooker, G. M. Chippendale, N. Hall, B. P. M. Hyland, R. D. Johnston, D. A. Kleinig, M. W. McDonald, and J. D. Turner. *Forest Trees of Australia.* 5th ed. Collingwood, Victoria, Australia: CSIRO Publishing, 2006.

Bonar, Ann. *The MacMillan Treasury of Herbs: A Complete Guide to the Cultivation and Use of Wild and Domesticated Herbs.* New York: MacMillan, 1985.

Brown, Kathleen. *Herbal Teas for Lifelong Health.* Recipe development by Jeanine Pollack. North Adams, MA: Storey Publishing, 1999.

Bruneau, Stephanie. *The Benevolent Bee: Capture the Bounty of the Hive Through Science, History, Home Remedies, and Craft.* Beverly, MA: Quarto Publishing Group USA, 2017.

Butler, Hilda, ed. *Poucher's Perfumes, Cosmetics and Soaps.* 10th ed. Dordrecht, The Netherlands: Springer Science+Business Media, 2000.

Campion, Kitty. *The Family Medical Herbal: A Complete Guide to Maintaining Health and Treating Illness with Plants.* New York: Barnes & Noble Books, 1996.

Castleman, Michael. *The New Healing Herbs: The Essential Guide to More than 130 of Nature's Most Potent Herbal Remedies.* 4th ed. Emmaus, PA: Rodale Press, 2010.

Centers for Disease Control and Prevention. "Prevent Mosquito Bites." List of insect repellents for mosquitoes registered with the EPA (Environmental Protection Agency). Accessed April 25, 2019. https://www.cdc.gov/zika/prevention/prevent-mosquito-bites.html.

Chandra, Anjana Motihar. *India Condensed: 5,000 Years of History and Culture.* Singapore: Marshall Cavendish Editions, 2008.

Chevallier, Andrew. *The Encyclopedia of Medicinal Plants: A Practical Reference Guide to Over 550 Key Herbs and Their Medicinal Uses.* New York: Dorling Kindersley Publishing, 1996.

———. *Herbal Remedies.* New York: Dorling Kindersley Publishing, 2007.

Clay, Horace F., and James C. Hubbard. *Tropical Shrubs.* Honolulu, HI: University Press of Hawaii, 1977.

Colonial Dames of America. *Herbs and Herb Lore of Colonial America.* New York: Dover Publications, 1995.

Coombes, Allen J. *Dictionary of Plant Names.* Portland, OR: Timber Press, 1985.

Couplan, François. *The Encyclopedia of Edible Plants of North America: Nature's Green Feast.* New Canaan, CT: Keats Publishing, 1998.

Cumo, Christopher. *Foods That Changed History: How Foods Shaped Civilization from the Ancient World to the Present.* Santa Barbara, CA: ABC-CLIO, 2015.

———, ed. *Encyclopedia of Cultivated Plants: From Acacia to Zinnia.* Vol. 3. Santa Barbara, CA: ABC-CLIO, 2013.

Dalby, Andrew. *Food in the Ancient World From A to Z.* New York: Routledge, 2003.

Damian, Peter, and Kate Damian. *Aromatherapy: Scent and Psyche: Using Essential Oils for Physical and Emotional Well-Being.* Rochester, VT: Healing Arts Press, 1995.

De la Tour, Shatoiya. *Earth Mother Herbal.* Gloucester, MA: Fair Winds, 2002.

Dugo, Giovanni, and Ivana Bonaccorsi, eds. *Citrus bergamia: Bergamot and Its Derivatives.* Boca Raton, FL: CRC Press, 2014.

Duke, James A. *Duke's Handbook of Medicinal Herbs.* 2nd ed. Boca Raton, FL: CRC Press, 2002.

———. *CRC Handbook of Medicinal Spices.* Boca Raton, FL: CRC Press, 2003.

———. *Duke's Handbook of Medicinal Plants of the Bible.* Boca Raton, FL: CRC Press, 2008.

———. *Duke's Handbook of Medicinal Plants of Latin America.* Boca Raton, FL: CRC Press, 2009.

Durkin, Philip. *The Oxford Guide to Etymology.* New York: Oxford University Press, 2009.

Farrer-Halls, Gill. *The Aromatherapy Bible: The Definitive Guide to Using Essential Oils.* New York: Sterling Publishing, 2005.

Felty, Sheryl L. *Grow 15 Herbs for the Kitchen.* North Adams, MA: Storey Publishing, 1981.

Fernie, William Thomas. *Herbal Simples: Approved for Modern Uses of Cure.* London: Simpkin, Marshall, Hamilton, Kent & Co., 1895.

Fischer-Rizzi, Susanne. *Complete Aromatherapy Handbook: Essential Oils for Radiant Health.* New York: Sterling Publishing, 1990.

Foster, Steven, and Rebecca L. Johnson. *National Geographic Desk Reference to Nature's Medicine.* Washington, DC: National Geographic Society, 2008.

Franck, Robert R., ed. *Bast and Other Plant Fibres.* Boca Raton, FL: CRC Press, 2005.

Fulder, Stephen, PhD, and John Blackwood. *Garlic: Nature's Original Remedy.* Rochester, VT: Healing Arts Press, 2000.

Gilbert, Avery. *What the Nose Knows: The Science of Scent in Everyday Life.* Fort Collins, CO: Synesthetics, 2014.

Goreja, W. G. *Shea Butter: The Nourishing Properties of Africa's Best-Kept Natural Beauty Secret.* New York: Amazing Herbs Press, 2004.

Govert, Johndennis. *Feng Shui: Art and Harmony of Place.* Phoenix: Daikakuji Publications, 1993.

Green, Aliza. *Field Guide to Herbs & Spices: How to Identify, Select, and Use Virtually Every Seasoning at the Market.* Philadelphia: Quirk Productions, 2006.

_____. *Field Guide to Produce: How to Identify, Select, and Prepare Virtually Every Fruit and Vegetable at the Market.* Philadelphia, PA: Quirk Productions, 2004.

Gregg, Susan. *The Complete Illustrated Encyclopedia of Magical Plants.* Beverly, MA: Fair Winds Press, 2008.

· · · · · · ·

Bibliography

Grieve, Maud. *A Modern Herbal*. 2 vols. New York: Dover Publications, 1971.

Groom, Nigel. *The New Perfume Handbook*. 2nd ed. London: Chapman & Hall, 1997.

Gut, Bernardo. *Trees in Patagonia*. Basel, Switzerland: Birkhäuser Verlag AG, 2008.

Halpern, Georges M. *The Healing Trail: Essential Oils of Madagascar*. North Bergen, NJ: Basic Health Publications, 2003.

Hanelt, Peter, and Institute of Plant Genetics and Crop Plant Research, eds. *Mansfeld's Encyclopedia of Agricultural and Horticultural Crops (Except Ornamentals)*. New York: Springer, 2001.

Harkness, Peter. *The Rose: An Illustrated History*. Buffalo, NY: Firefly Books, 2003.

Harrison, Lorraine. *Latin for Gardeners: Over 3,000 Plant Names Explained and Explored*. Chicago, IL: The University of Chicago Press, 2012.

Hatfield, Gabrielle. *Encyclopedia of Folk Medicine: Old World and New World Traditions*. Santa Barbara, CA: ABC-CLIO, 2004.

Heilmeyer, Marina. *Ancient Herbs*. Translated by David J. Baker. Los Angeles, CA: J. Paul Getty Museum, 2007.

Hibler, Janie. *The Berry Bible*. New York: William Morrow, 2004.

Higley, Connie, and Alan Higley. *Quick Reference Guide for Essential Oils*. 9th ed. Spanish Fork, UT: Abundant Health, 2005.

Holmes, Peter. *Aromatica: A Clinical Guide to Essential Oil Therapeutics*. Philadelphia, PA: Singing Dragon, 2016.

Insel, Paul, Don Ross, Kimberley McMahon, and Melissa Bernstein. *Discovering Nutrition*. 5th ed. Burlington, MA: Jones & Bartlett Learning, 2016.

Janardhanan, Minija, and John E. Thoppil. *Herb and Spice Essential Oils: Therapeutic, Flavour and Aromatic Chemicals of Apiaceae*. New Delhi, India: Discovery Publishing House, 2004.

Janick, Jules, and Robert E. Paull, eds. *The Encyclopedia of Fruit and Nuts*. Cambridge, MA: CABI North American Office, 2008.

Jones, Marlene. *The Complete Guide to Creating Oils, Soaps, Creams, and Herbal Gels for Your Mind and Body: 101 Natural Body Care Recipes*. Ocala, FL: Atlantic Publishing Group, 2011.

Jones, Peter C., and Lisa MacDonald, eds. *The Gardener's Almanac*. Boston, MA: Houghton Mifflin, 1997.

Jordan, E. Bernard. *The Laws of Thinking: 20 Secrets to Using the Divine Power of Your Mind to Manifest Prosperity*. Carlsbad, CA: Hay House, 2007.

Jünemann, Monika. *Enchanting Scents: The Secrets of Aroma Therapy*. Wilmot, WI: Lotus Light Publications, 1988.

· · · · · · ·

Kavasch, E. Barrie. *Medicine Wheel Garden: Creating Sacred Space for Healing, Celebration, and Tranquility.* New York: Bantam Books, 2002.

Khan, Iqrar Ahmad, ed. *Citrus Genetics, Breeding and Biotechnology.* Cambridge, MA: CABI, 2007.

Kiple, Kenneth F., and Kriemhild Coneè Ornelas, eds. *The Cambridge World History of Food.* Vols. 1 and 2. New York: Cambridge University Press, 2001.

Kowalchik, Claire, and William H. Hylton, eds. *Rodale's Illustrated Encyclopedia of Herbs.* Emmaus, PA: Rodale Press, 1998.

Kremers, Edward. *Kremers and Urdang's History of Pharmacy.* 4th ed. Revised by Glenn Sonnedecker. Philadelphia, PA: Lippincott, 1976.

Lane, Clive. *Plants for Small Spaces.* Boston, MA: Horticulture Books, 2005.

Langenheim, Jean H. *Plant Resins: Chemistry, Evolution, Ecology, and Ethnobotany.* Portland, OR: Timber Press, 2003.

Lavabre, Marcel F. *Aromatherapy Workbook.* Rochester, VT: Healing Arts Press, 1990.

Lawless, Julia. *The Complete Illustrated Guide to Aromatherapy: A Practical Approach to the Use of Essential Oils for Health and Well-Being.* London: Element Books, 1999.

_____. *The Illustrated Encyclopedia of Essential Oils: The Complete Guide to the Use of Oils in Aromatherapy and Herbalism.* London: Element Books, 1995.

Leland, Charles Godfrey. *Gypsy Sorcery and Fortune-telling.* London: T. Fisher Unwin, 1891.

Lowitz, Leza, and Reema Datta. *Sacred Sanskrit Words: For Yoga, Chant, and Meditation.* Berkeley, CA: Stone Bridge Press, 2005.

MacEwan, Peter, ed. *The Chemist and Druggist: A Weekly Journal of Pharmacy and the Drug Trade.* Vol. 39. London: The Chemist and Druggist, July 1891.

Mackenzie, Donald A. *Myths of China and Japan.* Whitefish, MT: Kessinger Publishing, 2005.

Martin, Ingrid. *Aromatherapy for Massage Practitioners.* Philadelphia, PA: Lippincott Williams & Wilkins, 2007.

McGovern, Patrick E., Stuart J. Fleming, and Solomon H. Katz, eds. *The Origins and Ancient History of Wine.* Amsterdam, The Netherlands: Gordon and Breach Publishers, 1996.

McKenna, Dennis J., Kenneth Jones, and Kerry Hughes. *Botanical Medicines: The Desk Reference for Major Herbal Supplements.* 2nd ed. New York: Routledge, 2011.

McLeod, Judyth A. *In a Unicorn's Garden: Recreating the Mystery and Magic of Medieval Gardens.* London: Murdoch Books, 2008.

McVicar, Jekka. *Grow Herbs: An Inspiring Guide to Growing and Using Herbs.* London: Dorling Kindersley, 2010.

· · · · · · ·

Bibliography

Michalun, M. Varinia, and Joseph C. DiNardo. *Milady Skin Care and Cosmetic Ingredients Dictionary.* 4th ed. Boston, MA: Cengage Learning, 2014.

Miller, Light, and Bryan Miller. *Ayurveda and Aromatherapy: The Earth Essential Guide to Ancient Wisdom and Modern Healing.* Twin Lakes, WI: Lotus Press, 1996.

Miller, Richard Alan, and Iona Miller. *The Magical and Ritual Use of Perfumes.* Rochester, VT: Destiny Books, 1990.

Moerman, Daniel E. *Native American Medicinal Plants: An Ethnobotanical Dictionary.* Portland, OR: Timber Press, 2009.

Mojay, Gabriel. *Aromatherapy for Healing the Spirit: Restoring Emotional and Mental Balance with Essential Oils.* Rochester, VT: Healing Arts Press, 1997.

Monaghan, Patricia. *The Encyclopedia of Celtic Mythology and Folklore.* New York: Facts On File, 2004.

Moody-Weis, Jennifer. "The Population Ecology of Sunflowers (Helianthus Annuus) Through Space and Time." PhD diss., University of Kansas, 2007. Ann Arbor, MI: Proquest Information & Learning Company. Accessed September 15, 2017, at http://www.proquest.com/products-services/dissertations.

Murray, Frank. *Health Benefits Derived from Sweet Orange: Diosmin Supplements from Citrus.* Laguna Beach, CA: Basic Health Publications, 2007.

Murray, Michael, Joseph Pizzorno, and Lara Pizzorno. *The Encyclopedia of Healing Foods.* New York: Atria Books, 2005.

Nandwani, Dilip, ed. *Sustainable Horticultural Systems: Issues, Technology and Innovation.* New York: Springer, 2014.

Neal, Bill. *Gardener's Latin: Discovering the Origins, Lore & Meanings of Botanical Names.* Chapel Hill, NC: Algonquin Books of Chapel Hill, 1992.

Nugent, Jeff, and Julia Boniface. *Permaculture Plants: A Selection.* White River Junction, VT: Chelsea Green Publishing, 2005.

Oxford Dictionary of English. 3rd ed. New York: Oxford University Press, 2010.

Panda, H. *Essential Oils Handbook.* Delhi, India: National Institute of Industrial Research, 2003.

Paull, Robert E., and Odilo Duarte. *Tropical Fruits.* Vol. 1. 2nd ed. Cambridge, MA: CABI, 2011.

Pauwels, Ivo, and Gerty Christoffels. *Herbs: Healthy Living with Herbs from Your Own Garden.* Cape Town, South Africa: Struik Publishers, 2006.

Peter, K. V., ed. *Handbook of Herbs and Spices.* Vol. 2. 2nd ed. Philadelphi, PA: Woodhead Publishing, 2004.

• • • • • • • •

Phaneuf, Holly. *Herbs Demystified: A Scientist Explains How the Most Common Herbal Remedies Really Work*. New York: Marlowe & Co., 2005.

Phillips, Steven J., Patricia Wentworth Comus, Mark A. Dimmitt, and Linda M. Brewer, eds. *A Natural History of the Sonoran Desert*. 2nd ed. Oakland, CA: University of California Press, 2015.

Pickles, Sheila, ed. *The Language of Flowers*. New York: Harmony Books, 1990.

Platt, Ellen Spector. *Lemon Herbs: How to Grow and Use 18 Great Plants*. Mechanicsburg, PA: Stackpole Books, 2002.

Pleasant, Barbara. *The Whole Herb: For Cooking, Crafts, Gardening, Health and Other Joys of Life*. Garden City Park, NY: Square One Publishers, 2004.

Poth, Susanne, and Gina Sauer. *The Spice Lilies: Eastern Secrets to Healing with Ginger, Turmeric, Cardamom, and Galangal*. Rochester, VT: Healing Arts Press, 2000.

Poucher, W. A. *Poucher's Perfumes, Cosmetics and Soaps: The Production, Manufacture and Application of Perfumes*. Vol. 2. 9th ed. New York: Chapman & Hall, 1997.

Prance, Sir Ghillean, and Mark Nesbitt, eds. *The Cultural History of Plants*. New York: Routledge, 2005.

Price, Shirley. *Aromatherapy for Common Ailments*. New York: Fireside, 1991.

Quattrocchi, Umberto. *CRC World Dictionary of Plant Names: Common Names, Scientific Names, Eponyms, Synonyms, and Etymology*. Vol. 1. Boca Raton, FL: CRC Press, 2016.

Raghavan, Susheela. *Handbook of Spices, Seasonings, and Flavorings*. 2nd ed. Boca Raton, FL: CRC Press, 2007.

Ransome, Hilda M. *The Sacred Bee in Ancient Times and Folklore*. Mineola, NY: Dover Publications, 2004. First published 1937.

Raven, Peter H., Ray F. Evert, and Susan E. Eichhorn. *Biology of Plants*. 7th ed. New York: W. H. Freeman and Co., 2005.

Rayburn, Debra. *Let's Get Natural with Herbs*. Huntsville, AR: Ozark Mountain Publishing, 2007.

Reader's Digest, ed. *Magic and Medicine of Plants*. Pleasantville, NY: Reader's Digest Association, 1986.

Ridley, Henry Nicholas. *Spices*. London: Macmillan and Co., 1912.

Rieger, Mark. *Introduction to Fruit Crops*. Binghamton, NY: Food Products Press, 2006.

Roberts, Margaret. *Edible & Medicinal Flowers*. Claremont, South Africa: The Spearhead Press, 2007.

Rodd, Tony, and Jennifer Stackhouse. *Trees: A Visual Guide*. Berkeley, CA: University of California Press, 2008.

• • • • • • •

Bibliography

Rogers, Juliette. *Grow 15 Herbs for Fragrance.* North Adams, MA: Storey Publishing, 1999.

Rose, Jeanne. *Herbs & Things: Jeanne Rose's Herbal.* San Francisco, CA: Last Gasp of San Francisco, 2005.

_____. *375 Essential Oils and Hydrosols.* Berkeley, CA: Frog, 1999.

Rosengarten, Frederic, Jr. *The Book of Edible Nuts.* Mineola, NY: Dover Publications, 2004.

Santerre, Charles R., ed. *Pecan Technology.* New York: Chapman & Hall, 1994.

Sauer, Jonathan D. *Historical Geography of Crop Plants: A Select Roster.* Boca Raton, FL: CRC Press, 1993.

Schiller, Carol, and David Schiller. *The Aromatherapy Encyclopedia: A Concise Guide to Over 385 Plant Oils.* Laguna Beach, CA: Basic Health Publications, 2008.

_____. *500 Formulas for Aromatherapy: Mixing Essential Oils for Every Use.* New York: Sterling Publishing, 1994.

Seidemann, Johannes. *World Spice Plants: Economic Usage, Botany, Taxonomy.* New York: Springer-Verlag, 2005.

Sell, Charles S., ed. *The Chemistry of Fragrances: From Perfumer to Consumer.* 2nd ed. Cambridge, England: Royal Society of Chemistry, 2006.

Seymour, Miranda. *A Brief History of Thyme and Other Herbs.* New York: Grove Press, 2002.

Small, Ernest. *Top 100 Food Plants: The World's Most Important Culinary Crops.* Ottawa, Canada: NCR Research Press, 2009.

Small, Ernest, and Paul M. Catling. *Canadian Medicinal Crops.* Ottawa, Canada: National Research Council of Canada, 1999.

Sonneman, Toby. *Lemon: A Global History.* London: Reaktion Books, 2012.

Southwell, Ian, and Robert Lowe, eds. *Tea Tree: The Genus Melaleuca.* Amsterdam, The Netherlands: Hardwood Academic Publishers, 2005.

Staub, Jack. *75 Exceptional Herbs for Your Garden.* Layton, UT: Gibbs Smith, 2008.

_____. *75 Remarkable Fruits for Your Garden.* Layton, UT: Gibbs Smith, 2007.

Steel, Susannah, ed. *Home Herbal: Cook, Brew & Blend Your Own Herbs.* New York: Dorling Kindersley Publishing, 2011.

Stokes, Dustin, Mohan Matthen, and Stephen Biggs, eds. *Perception and Its Modalities.* New York: Oxford University Press, 2015.

Tisserand, Robert, and Rodney Young. *Essential Oil Safety: A Guide for Health Care Professionals.* 2nd ed. New York: Churchill Livingstone, 2014.

Toussaint-Samat, Maguelonne. *A History of Food.* Translated from the French by Anthea Bell. Malden, MA: John Wiley & Sons, 2009.

· · · · · · ·

Tucker, Arthur O., and Thomas DeBaggio. *The Encyclopedia of Herbs: A Comprehensive Reference to Herbs of Flavor and Fragrance*. Portland, OR: Timber Press, 2009.

Van Wyk, Ben-Erik, and Michael Wink. *Medicinal Plants of the World*. Portland, OR: Timber Press, 2004.

Visser, Margaret. *Much Depends on Dinner: The Extraordinary History and Mythology, Allure and Obsessions, Perils and Taboos, of an Ordinary Meal*. New York: Grove Press, 1986.

Warrier, P. K., V. P. K. Nambiar, and C. Ramankutty, eds. *Indian Medicinal Plants: A Compendium of 500 Species*. Vol. 2. Chennai, India: Orient Longman, 2005.

Watson, Franzesca. *Aromatherapy Blends and Remedies*. London: Thorsons, 1995.

Watts, Donald. *Elsevier's Dictionary of Plant Lore*. Burlington, MA: Academic Press, 2007.

Webster's II New College Dictionary. 3rd ed. New York: Houghton Mifflin, 2005.

Webster's Third New International Dictionary of the English Language, Unabridged. Springfield, MA: G. & C. Merriam Co., 1981.

Weiss, E. A. *Spice Crops*. New York: CABI Publishing, 2002.

Wells, Diana. *Lives of the Trees: An Uncommon History*. Chapel Hill, NC: Algonquin Books of Chapel Hill, 2010.

Wheelwright, Edith Grey. *Medicinal Plants and Their History*. New York: Dover Publications, 1974.

Williams, Cheryll J. *Medicinal Plants in Australia, Vol. 2: Gums, Resins, Tannin and Essential Oils*. Kenthurst, Australia: Rosenberg Publishing, 2011.

Wilson, Roberta. *Aromatherapy: Essential Oils for Vibrant Health and Beauty*. New York: Avery, 2002.

Wood, Matthew. *Earthwise Herbal: A Complete Guide to Old World Medicinal Plants*. Berkeley, CA: North Atlantic Books, 2008.

Worwood, Susan, and Valerie Ann Worwood. *Essential Aromatherapy: A Pocket Guide to Essential Oils and Aromatherapy*. Novato, CA: New World Library, 2003.

Worwood, Valerie Ann. *The Complete Book of Essential Oils and Aromatherapy*. Novato, CA: New World Library, 1991.

Zak, Victoria. *The Magic Teaspoon: Transform Your Meals with the Power of Healing Herbs and Spices*. New York: Berkley Books, 2006.

Zohary, Daniel, Maria Hopf, and Ehud Weiss. *Domestication of Plants in the Old World*. 4th ed. New York: Oxford University Press, 2012.

• • • • • • •

INDEX

· · · · · · ·

• • • • • • •

• • • • • • •

• • • • • • •

• • • • • • •

• • • • • • •

• • • • • • •

R

S

· · · · · · ·

To Write to the Author

If you wish to contact the author or would like more information about this book, please write to the author in care of Llewellyn Worldwide Ltd. and we will forward your request. Both the author and the publisher appreciate hearing from you and learning of your enjoyment of this book and how it has helped you. Llewellyn Worldwide Ltd. cannot guarantee that every letter written to the author can be answered, but all will be forwarded. Please write to:

Sandra Kynes
℅ Llewellyn Worldwide
2143 Wooddale Drive
Woodbury, MN 55125-2989

Please enclose a self-addressed stamped envelope for reply,
or $1.00 to cover costs. If outside the U.S.A., enclose
an international postal reply coupon.

Many of Llewellyn's authors have websites with additional information and resources.

For more information, please visit our website at http://www.llewellyn.com.

GET MORE AT LLEWELLYN.COM

Visit us online to browse hundreds of our books and decks, plus sign up to receive our e-newsletters and exclusive online offers.

- **Free tarot readings** • **Spell-a-Day** • **Moon phases**
- **Recipes, spells, and tips** • **Blogs** • **Encyclopedia**
- **Author interviews, articles, and upcoming events**

GET SOCIAL WITH LLEWELLYN

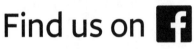

Find us on

@LlewellynBooks

www.Facebook.com/LlewellynBooks

GET BOOKS AT LLEWELLYN

LLEWELLYN ORDERING INFORMATION

Order online: Visit our website at www.llewellyn.com to select your books and place an order on our secure server.

Order by phone:
- Call toll free within the US at 1-877-NEW-WRLD (1-877-639-9753)
- We accept VISA, MasterCard, American Express, and Discover.

Order by mail:
Send the full price of your order (MN residents add 6.875% sales tax) in US funds plus postage and handling to: Llewellyn Worldwide, 2143 Wooddale Drive, Woodbury, MN 55125-2989

POSTAGE AND HANDLING

STANDARD (US):(Please allow 12 business days)
$30.00 and under, add $6.00.
$30.01 and over, FREE SHIPPING.

CANADA:
We cannot ship to Canada. Please shop your local bookstore or Amazon Canada.

INTERNATIONAL:
Customers pay the actual shipping cost to the final destination, which includes tracking information.

Visit us online for more shipping options. Prices subject to change.

FREE CATALOG!

To order, call
1-877-
NEW-WRLD
ext. 8236
or visit our
website

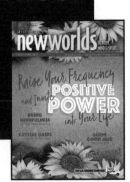

"Highly recommended to anyone who has an interest in aromatherapy and the energetic and vibrational aspects of essential oils." —KELLY HOLLAND AZZARO, Past President of the National Association for Holistic Aromatherapy

THE
HEALING
ART
OF
ESSENTIAL
OILS

**A GUIDE TO 50 OILS FOR
REMEDY, RITUAL, AND EVERYDAY USE**

KAC YOUNG, PhD

The Healing Art of Essential Oils
A Guide to 50 Oils for Remedy, Ritual, and Everyday Use
Kac Young, PhD

Explore a new world of aromatic awakening, physical healing, and natural delight. *The Healing Art of Essential Oils* is a comprehensive guide to fifty carefully selected oils, providing a master class in uses, blending, history, and spiritual benefits.

Learn how to use oils for physical and emotional healing. Prepare oils for relaxation, stress relief, and treating ailments. You'll find all kinds of uses, such as what oils work best in love spells and how to create rituals with oils. Enjoyed for their spiritual and beneficial properties by cultures around the world for thousands of years, the essential oils presented here will help you achieve holistic wellness and personal enrichment.

978-0-7387-5047-7, 384 pp., 7 ½ x 9 ¼ $21.99

To order, call 1-877-NEW-WRLD or visit llewellyn.com
Prices subject to change without notice

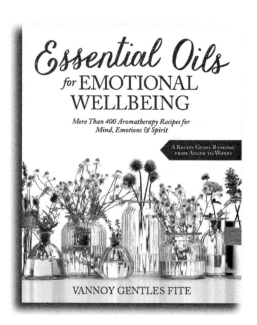

Essential Oils for Emotional Wellbeing
More Than 400 Aromatherapy Recipes for Mind, Emotions & Spirit
Vannoy Gentles Fite

Throughout the ages, essential oils have been used to address a wide variety of mental, emotional, and spiritual needs. Bring this ancient knowledge into your modern life with *Essential Oils for Emotional Wellbeing*. Featuring more than 400 step-by-step recipes, this comprehensive guide makes it easy for you to take control of your wellness and spiritual journey. These recipes come in many forms, including:

- Bath and shower bombs
- Bath salts
- Lotions
- Ointments
- Diffuser scents
- Powders
- Rubs
- Salves
- Sprays
- Lip balms
- Massage oils
- Inhalants

It's simple to find the recipes you need with this book's well-organized categories based on conditions, emotions, needs, desires, and devotion. Learn about therapeutic properties, warnings, storage, and using essential oils for specific issues. With Vannoy Gentles Fite's guidance, you'll be able to use these gifts from the earth to benefit every aspect of your life.

978-0-7387-5663-9, 432 pp., 7 ½ x 9 ¼ $37.99

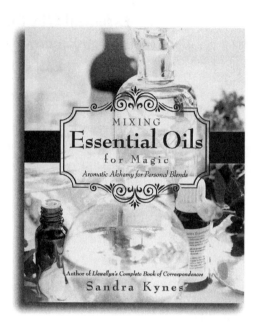

MIXING
Essential Oils
for Magic
Aromatic Alchemy for Personal Blends

Author of *Llewellyn's Complete Book of Correspondences*
Sandra Kynes

Mixing Essential Oils for Magic
Aromatic Alchemy for Personal Blends
SANDRA KYNES

This straightforward guide will help you understand how to choose the best oils for your own creative and magical mixing. Not only will you find step-by-step instructions on how to measure, mix, and assess blends, but you will also gain a full understanding of essential and carrier oils and how they work together.

Mixing Essential Oils for Magic is divided into three sections: the historical background of oils and their present-day uses, an encyclopedic listing of plant profiles from which essential and carrier oils come, and thorough cross-references for the oils and their magical associations. Learn about the historical uses of scent in ritual, how to blend oils by botanical family, scent group, perfume note, or magical association, and also how to make unique mixes an integral part of your spiritual and magical practices.

978-0-7387-3654-9, 336 pp., 7½ x 9⅛   **$21.99**

To order, call 1-877-NEW-WRLD or visit llewellyn.com
Prices subject to change without notice

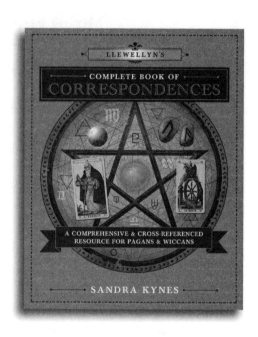

LLEWELLYN'S

COMPLETE BOOK OF

CORRESPONDENCES

A COMPREHENSIVE & CROSS-REFERENCED
RESOURCE FOR PAGANS & WICCANS

SANDRA KYNES

Llewellyn's Complete Book of Correspondences
A Comprehensive & Cross-Referenced Resource for Pagans & Wiccans
Sandra Kynes

Llewellyn's Complete Book of Correspondences is a clear, straightforward companion to the many books on Wiccan and Pagan ritual and spellwork. Entries are cross-referenced and indexed, and organized by categories and subcategories, making it quick and easy to find what you need.

This comprehensive reference provides a fascinating look at why correspondences are more than objects to focus intent, but are fundamental to how we think. Using correspondences weaves together our ideas, beliefs, and energy, and gives deeper meaning to our rituals and spellwork as we unite our individuality with a larger purpose.

Packed with content yet easy to use, this book covers traditional correspondences and also encourages you to forge new ones that hold special meaning for you.

978-0-7387-3253-4, 552 pp., 8 x 10　　　　　　　　　　　　　　　　　　　　$34.99

To order, call 1-877-NEW-WRLD or visit llewellyn.com
Prices subject to change without notice

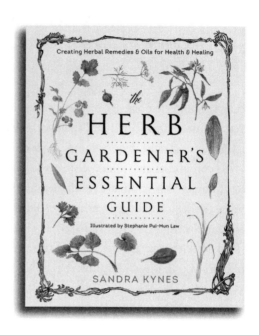

Creating Herbal Remedies & Oils for Health & Healing

the

HERB
GARDENER'S
ESSENTIAL
GUIDE

Illustrated by Stephanie Pui-Mun Law

SANDRA KYNES

The Herb Gardener's Essential Guide
Creating Herbal Remedies and Oils for Health & Healing
SANDRA KYNES

Learn how to use twenty-eight popular, easy-to-grow herbs to treat everyday ailments and maintain good health. From selecting plants to harvesting and storing them to making remedies and savories of all sorts, *The Herb Gardener's Essential Guide* presents an abundance of practical and satisfying ways to incorporate herbs into a healthier lifestyle and diet.

Utilizing both herbs and essential oils, this beautifully illustrated guide explains how to choose and make the ideal herbal mixture for a wide variety of medicinal and culinary uses. Need help getting to sleep? Try a cup of Thyme to Settle Tea. Add a sweet, spicy flavor to roast meat or vegetables with Coriander Spiced Butter. Ease muscle pain and stiffness with soothing Rosemary Warming Massage Oil. Featuring an ailments-and-issues guide, instructions for creating a personalized apothecary garden, and detailed profiles for each of the herbs, this accessible book belongs on every gardener's shelf.

978-0-7387-4564-0, 264 pp., 8 x 10   **$22.99**

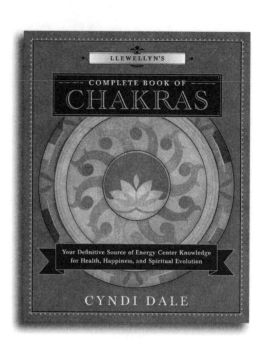

LLEWELLYN'S

COMPLETE BOOK OF

CHAKRAS

Your Definitive Source of Energy Center Knowledge
for Health, Happiness, and Spiritual Evolution

CYNDI DALE

Llewellyn's Complete Book of Chakras
Your Definitive Source of Energy Center Knowledge
for Health, Happiness, and Spiritual Evolution
CYNDI DALE

As powerful centers of subtle energy, the chakras have fascinated humanity for thousands of years. *Llewellyn's Complete Book of Chakras* is a unique and empowering resource that provides comprehensive insights into these foundational sources of vitality and strength. Discover what chakras and chakra systems are, how to work with them for personal growth and healing, and the ways our understanding of chakras has transformed throughout time and across cultures.

Lively and accessible, this definitive reference explores the science, history, practices, and structures of our subtle energy. With an abundance of illustrations and a wealth of practical exercises, Cyndi Dale shows you how to use chakras for improving wellness, attracting what you need, obtaining guidance, and expanding your consciousness.

978-0-7387-3962-5, 1,056 pp., 8 x 10 $44.99

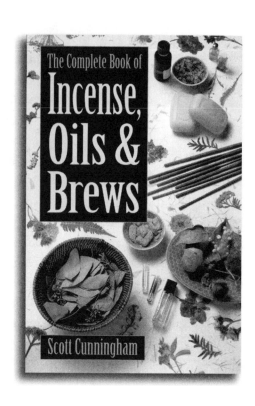

The Complete Book of
Incense, Oils & Brews

Scott Cunningham

The Complete Book of Incense, Oils & Brews
Scott Cunningham

One of the secrets of real magic is that it is controlled by the mind. The more things in your ritual to help your mind associate with your goal, the more powerful your ritual may be. Colored candles, scented oils, natural incenses, and more all add to the impact of the magic you wish to do. But how do you know which incense to burn? Is it possible to add scented oils together to get a more powerful oil? And how do you make your own appropriately scented tools?

The answers to questions like these and hundreds more can be found in *The Complete Book of Incense, Oils & Brews* by world-famous author Scott Cunningham. This is a greatly expanded and rewritten version of *The Magic of Incenses, Oils & Brews*. It includes over 100 new formulas, proportions for each element of the recipes (the most requested feature from his previous book), how to substitute ingredients, and much more. Besides the formulas, it also includes the exact methods of making all of these scented tools, including how to extract the essences from the herbs.

Each one of the formulas in this magic book is precise and easy to make. Do you need luck? Take 2 parts vetivert, 2 parts allspice, 1 part nutmeg, and 1 part calamus, grind them together as finely as possible, then sprinkle the powder in a circle around you, beginning and ending in the east and moving clockwise. Sit within this circle and absorb the powder's energies. Also included are other ways to use magical powders that will have you coming up with your own ideas for them, too.

There is a legion of recipes for incenses. There are three for the sun and two for consecrating talismans. There are incenses for each of the astrological signs and ones to help you study better and gain success. You'll also find incenses for each of the planetary influences. There are four for Saturn alone!

This compendium of magical lore is a vital tool for every magical person on any magical path, whether you are a beginner or an expert.

978-0-87542-128-5, 288 pp., 6 x 9   **$17.99**

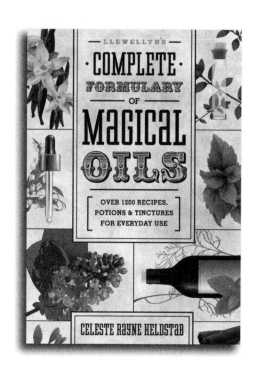

Llewellyn's Complete Formulary of Magical Oils
Over 1200 Recipes, Potions & Tinctures for Everyday Use
CELESTE RAYNE HELDSTAB

Step into the fantastically fragrant world of magical oils and discover a new, invigorating way to delight your senses, uplift your spirits, improve your health, and enjoy total relaxation. Whether your intention is magical or medicinal, specially blended essential oils can enrich your life with their mystical, energizing, and transformative power.

Within this one-of-a-kind portable apothecary, learn to select and mix 67 essential oils for a myriad of magical, medicinal, and spiritual applications. Spanning every purpose from inner calm and romance to healing and energy work to prayer and spellcraft, all 1,200 recipes are arranged alphabetically to make it easy to find precisely what you need.

Step by step, Celeste Rayne Heldstab also shows how to create your own blends for spells, rituals, and remedies. Amp up their potency with correspondences for the elements, day of the week, time of day, moon phase, astrological sign, herbs, and gemstones.

- Protection for house and home
- Love and passion
- Career and finances
- Dreamwork and meditation
- Beauty and skin care
- Fatigue, headaches, and other common ailments

978-0-7387-2751-6, 432 pp., 7 x 10 $29.99

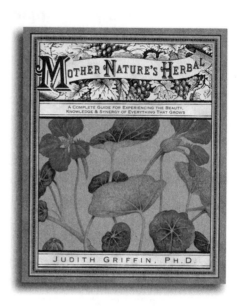

MOTHER NATURE'S HERBAL

A COMPLETE GUIDE FOR EXPERIENCING THE BEAUTY,
KNOWLEDGE & SYNERGY OF EVERYTHING THAT GROWS

JUDITH GRIFFIN, PH.D.

Mother Nature's Herbal
A Complete Guide for Experiencing the Beauty, Knowledge & Synergy of Everything That Grows
JUDITH GRIFFIN

Due to overwhelming demand since its debut ten years ago, this beloved guide to the herbal wisdom of Mother Nature is back! With ancient folklore, simple instructions for growing an herb garden, and recipes from around the world, *Mother Nature's Herbal* is hands down the most unique, thoughtful, and comprehensive guide to growing and preparing herbs.

Divided into useful sections and graced with charming illustrations, this book is the perfect addition to any budding herbalist's kitchen counter. Part one presents a rich tapestry of centuries-old customs, recipes, and mythology from various cultures, including Native American, South American, Asian, Mediterranean, medieval, colonial, and more.

Part two explains how to grow and use your own organic herbs. Make them thrive with tips on tending the soil, guarding against pests, and keeping your plants healthy. Once you've harvested your herbs, experiment with an assortment of recipes for foods, teas, tonics, ointments, and medicines. Explore the magical benefits of herbs, and enjoy invigorated health and a rejuvenated spirit!

978-0-7387-1256-7, 432 pp., 7½ x 9 3/16   **$29.99**

To order, call 1-877-NEW-WRLD or visit llewellyn.com
Prices subject to change without notice